Breaking Point

Breaking Point

Job Stress, Occupational Depression, and the Myth of Burnout

Irvin Sam Schonfeld, Ph.D., M.P.H.
The City College and the Graduate Center of the City University of New York

and

Renzo Bianchi, Ph.D.
Norwegian University of Science and Technology (NTNU)
WorkWell Research Unit, North-West University

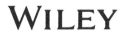

Copyright © 2025 by John Wiley and Sons, Inc. All rights reserved, including rights for text and data mining and training of artificial intelligence technologies or similar technologies

Published by John Wiley & Sons, Inc., Hoboken, New Jersey.
Published simultaneously in Canada.

No part of this publication may be reproduced, stored in a retrieval system, or transmitted in any form or by any means, electronic, mechanical, photocopying, recording, scanning, or otherwise, except as permitted under Section 107 or 108 of the 1976 United States Copyright Act, without either the prior written permission of the Publisher, or authorization through payment of the appropriate per-copy fee to the Copyright Clearance Center, Inc., 222 Rosewood Drive, Danvers, MA 01923, (978) 750–8400, fax (978) 750–4470, or on the web at www.copyright.com. Requests to the Publisher for permission should be addressed to the Permissions Department, John Wiley & Sons, Inc., 111 River Street, Hoboken, NJ 07030, (201) 748–6011, fax (201) 748–6008, or online at http://www.wiley.com/go/permission.

The manufacturer's authorized representative according to the EU General Product Safety Regulation is Wiley-VCH GmbH, Boschstr. 12, 69469 Weinheim, Germany, e-mail: Product_Safety@wiley.com.

Trademarks: Wiley and the Wiley logo are trademarks or registered trademarks of John Wiley & Sons, Inc. and/or its affiliates in the United States and other countries and may not be used without written permission. All other trademarks are the property of their respective owners. John Wiley & Sons, Inc. is not associated with any product or vendor mentioned in this book.

Limit of Liability/Disclaimer of Warranty: While the publisher and author have used their best efforts in preparing this book, they make no representations or warranties with respect to the accuracy or completeness of the contents of this book and specifically disclaim any implied warranties of merchantability or fitness for a particular purpose. No warranty may be created or extended by sales representatives or written sales materials. The advice and strategies contained herein may not be suitable for your situation. You should consult with a professional where appropriate. Further, readers should be aware that websites listed in this work may have changed or disappeared between when this work was written and when it is read. Neither the publisher nor authors shall be liable for any loss of profit or any other commercial damages, including but not limited to special, incidental, consequential, or other damages.

For general information on our other products and services or for technical support, please contact our Customer Care Department within the United States at (800) 762–2974, outside the United States at (317) 572–3993 or fax (317) 572–4002.

Wiley also publishes its books in a variety of electronic formats. Some content that appears in print may not be available in electronic formats. For more information about Wiley products, visit our web site at www.wiley.com.

Library of Congress Cataloging-in-Publication Data has been applied for.

Paperback: 9781394249497
ePDF: 9781394249527
ePub: 9781394249503
oBook: 9781394249626

Cover Design: Wiley
Cover Image: © crizzystudio/stock.adobe.com

Set in 9.5/12.5pts STIXTwo by Lumina Datamatics

For my wife, Pearl Knopf Schonfeld

And

In memory of my sister, Royce Joy Schonfeld Katsir
—**Irvin Sam Schonfeld**

Contents

Foreword *xi*
About the Authors *xiii*
Preface *xv*

1 Occupational Depression *1*
  Brief History of Depression *1*
  "Depression is rage turned inward," Dr. Jennifer Melfi *5*
  Challenge to Freud's Explanation of Depression *6*
  Helplessness and Hopelessness *10*
  Early Linkages of Work to Psychological State *11*
  The Diagnosis of Depression *15*
  Another Way to Think About Depression *17*
  Assessing Depression in the Research Context *19*
  "The Stress of Life" *19*
  Stressful Life Events *21*
  The Demand–Control (DC) Model of Job Stress *27*
  A New Development: The Demand–Control–Support (DCS) Model of Job Stress *32*
  Reverse Causality *33*
  The Effort–Reward Imbalance (ERI) Model *45*
  Workplace Bullying *47*
  Underestimates *53*
  Conclusions *55*
  Postscript *56*
  References *57*

2 **Burnout** 73
  Herbert J. Freudenberger 74
  Christina Maslach 76
  Correlation Coefficients and Reliability Coefficients 78
  The Foundations of Burnout 80
  More on Discriminant Validity 87
  Antecedents of Burnout 88
  The Multiplication of Burnout Scales 89
  Problems with Burnout Symptom Items That Are Synonymous 92
  Burnout as a Diagnosis 93
  Longitudinal Research on Adverse Working Conditions and Burnout 94
  Conclusions 103
  References 104

3 **Burnout-Depression Overlap** 111
  The Idea of a Syndrome 113
  First Look at Burnout-Depression Overlap 113
  Burnout and Depression as Distinct Constructs 114
  A Line of Research by Bianchi, Schonfeld, and Colleagues 116
  Burnout and Depressive Cognition 121
  Neurobiology of Burnout and Depression 123
  Anxiety and Depressive Symptoms 124
  The Occupational Depression Inventory 127
  Other Studies That Bear on Burnout-Depression Overlap 131
  Meta-analyses 133
  Conclusions 137
  References 141

4 **The Stigma Attached to Burnout** 153
  Some Background Beliefs 154
  What Empirical Research Indicates 155
  Burnout Versus Depression 156
  Destigmatizing Burnout 159
  Conclusions 160
  References 161

5 Interventions *165*

Models of Interventions *165*
Randomized Control Trials and Meta-analyses *168*
Tertiary Interventions *173*
Primary and Secondary Interventions for Depression, Psychological Distress, and Burnout *182*
A Pertinent Primary Intervention Study *189*
Conclusions *191*
References *194*

Appendix *203*
Occupational Depression Inventory (ODI) *203*
Inventaire de Dépression Professionnelle (IDP) *205*

Index *209*

Foreword

Breaking Point: Job Stress, Occupational Depression, and the Myth of Burnout by Irvin Sam Schonfeld and Renzo Bianchi is a groundbreaking exploration that challenges conventional wisdom about burnout and depression. The authors take readers on an enlightening journey through the history of depression, from its ancient roots to its modern understanding in psychiatry. They meticulously dissect the concept of burnout, revealing its deep connections to depressive disorders. Through their own rigorous research and the work of many other well-recognized colleagues in the field, the authors demonstrate that what is often labeled as burnout is, in fact, a manifestation of (occupational) depression.

The book is structured into five insightful chapters, each building on the last to create a comprehensive narrative. The authors begin by tracing the historical context of depression and its links to adverse working conditions. They then scrutinize the construct of burnout, highlighting its overlap with depression. The third chapter is a breaking point, presenting robust evidence of the burnout–depression overlap, supported by the authors' extensive research. The discussion on stigma and the need for destigmatization of mental health issues is both timely, crucial, and surprising even to scholars like me. Finally, the book offers practical interventions to help affected workers and improve working conditions, aiming to prevent job-related depression.

Breaking Point is not just a scholarly work; it is a call to action. Schonfeld and Bianchi's eloquent prose and compelling arguments make this book a must-read for professionals and laypersons alike. It challenges readers to rethink their understanding of burnout and depression, urging them to recognize the profound impact of job stress on mental health. This book is an essential addition to the conversation on workplace well-being, offering new perspectives and solutions to a critical issue.

Christian Dormann
Professor, Business Education & Management
Johannes Gutenberg-Universität Mainz

About the Authors

Irvin Sam Schonfeld, professor emeritus at The City College and the Graduate Center of the City University of New York, has studied the impact of job stress on workers, particularly teachers. He and Renzo Bianchi codeveloped the Occupational Depression Inventory and have worked to validate the instruments in several countries and languages. We have also codeveloped a second job-related instrument, the Occupational Anxiety Inventory. Other research interests include burnout–depression overlap, stress in the self-employed, multilevel modeling, and the interface of qualitative and quantitative research. He won an award from the Society for Occupational Health Psychology for his distinguished contribution to the field of occupational health psychology. He is also working on a memoir about growing up in a Brooklyn housing project.

Renzo Bianchi earned his doctoral degree in psychology from Bourgogne Franche-Comté University in 2014. After seven years as a lecturer and researcher at the University of Neuchâtel, with occasional academic duties at the University of Geneva, he joined the Norwegian University of Science and Technology (NTNU) as an associate professor of psychology in 2022. At NTNU, Renzo leads the MAD-OHP research group, which focuses on occupational health and psychological assessment. He is the co-creator of the Occupational Depression Inventory and the Occupational Anxiety Inventory. Since 2024, Renzo has additionally served as an extraordinary professor at the WorkWell Research Unit at North-West University. Renzo has (co-)authored over 100 scientific publications to date.

Preface

Our book has a prehistory that begins in 1991. In that year, Irvin was preparing two separate papers for national conferences, one on depression in teachers, and the other on burnout in teachers. He decided, based on his conference talks, to publish a short paper suggesting that there is more overlap between burnout and depression than many researchers suspected at that time. He published the paper in the database run by the Education Resources Information Center, better known by the acronym ERIC (Schonfeld, 1991).[1] The ERIC paper did not get much play. Irvin estimated that if he were to include his wife and sister, he could safely say that three people in the world read the paper. He was soon diverted away from questions relating to burnout and depression. With one exception, other research questions called for his attention, and he did not follow up on the ERIC paper. The exception was that a University of Maryland professor whom he met at a conference colloquium asked him to write a chapter on burnout and depression for a book about stress. The Maryland professor was the book's editor. Although Irvin wrote the chapter, unfortunately, it never got published because the publisher went out of business.

Twenty-one years after the ERIC paper was published, in December 2012, Irvin received an email from the editor of the *Journal of Health Psychology*. The editor asked him to review a submission. It was a time of year otherwise crowded with deadlines. Irvin was swamped with student papers to read, exams to mark, and grades to enter. And he and his

---

[1] Schonfeld, I. S. (1991). Burnout in teachers: Is it burnout or is it depression? ERIC Document No. 335329. http://www.eric.ed.gov/PDFS/ED335329.pdf

wife were planning their annual New Year's Day party. To lure reviewers, editors include an abstract of the manuscript up for review. Typically, during the reviewing process, the identities of submitters and reviewers are masked. Because he found the abstract tantalizing, awakening an interest in a subject he thought about many years earlier, he agreed to review the submission. The paper concerned three groups of French participants, a group of schoolteachers who had scores on the Maslach Burnout Inventory (MBI) that were relatively low, a group of teachers with relatively high scores on the MBI, and a group of depressed outpatients. Irvin found interesting that the depressive symptom profiles of the patients and the teachers with high burnout scores were largely similar and those two sets of symptom profiles dramatically differed from that of the teachers having low burnout scores. Irvin suggested that the authors make some small adjustments but recommended that the editor publish the paper.

After Irvin submitted his review to the editor, the month of December passed into January and January into February. He had forgotten about the paper he reviewed. Then in March 2013, he received an email from a French graduate student he did not know. The graduate student asked Irvin to collaborate on a research project. Irvin was busy and took time to think about the wording of a return-email to politely decline the graduate student's request without hurting the student's feelings.

Before he drafted that return email, he received a second email from the graduate student. Attached to the email was a PDF. To Irvin's surprise, the PDF contained an updated version of the paper he reviewed back in December. The paper had been accepted for publication.[2] The graduate student was Renzo. The paper demonstrated Renzo's *bona fides*. To Irvin, Renzo was the Real McCoy. Irvin agreed to collaborate with Renzo. That would be the beginning of a collaboration that has endured more than a decade.

Irvin knew that he was scheduled to spend a few days in Paris in July 2013, before traveling to Ferrara, Italy, to see an old friend. Renzo was still at his university in Besançon. The two of us arranged to meet in person in Paris and work on an ambitious paper on burnout–depression overlap.

---

2 Bianchi, R., Boffy, C., Hingray, C., Truchot, D., & Laurent, E. (2013). Comparative symptomatology of burnout and depression. *Journal of Health Psychology*, *18*(6), 782–787. https://doi.org/10.1177/1359105313481079

Éric Laurent, a professor at Bourgogne Franche-Comté University, the institution that in 2014 would award Renzo a doctorate, also contributed to that paper. Also in 2014, the *International Journal of Stress Management* published the paper.[3] The Journals Office of the American Psychological Association wrote to tell us that the paper received a great deal of interest on the APA's Facebook site, and the paper was spotlighted by the APA Center for Organizational Excellence. We knew we were onto something important. We rapidly published several additional papers.

We saw each other in person again in July 2015, in Besançon. During that visit, Irvin got to see some of the sites in eastern France and the *Suisse romande* (e.g., *la Citadelle*, the homes of Victor Hugo and the Lumiere brothers, and the Collegiate Church in Neuchâtel). Renzo and Irvin, however, spent considerable time drafting a proposal to CUNY's human subjects committee, seeking approval for a study they were planning to run in the United States. That human-subjects proposal eventually led to a study of burnout and depression that was published in the *Journal of Clinical Psychology* in 2016.[4] We were making progress.

We have thus been research collaborators since 2013. We have dedicated countless hours of work to clarify the burnout case, trying to address the issue as comprehensively as we could. Our work has resulted in dozens of studies and papers over the years. We are grateful for the sustained interest that our research has elicited not only among the scientific and medical communities but also among organizations and the public.

In the spring of 2023, Irvin received a request from an editor at John Wiley, asking him to review another author's book proposal about burnout. He read the proposal and wrote what he thought was a fair and thorough review. Some weeks after he sent the review to the editor, he received another email from the editor. In this email the editor asked Irvin to submit his own book proposal. Irvin asked Renzo if he would be willing to be a partner in writing the proposal and, if the proposal were accepted, to coauthor the proposed book. Upon Renzo's agreeing, Irvin

---

3 Bianchi, R., Schonfeld, I. S., & Laurent, E. (2014). Is burnout a depressive disorder? A reexamination with special focus on atypical depression. *International Journal of Stress Management, 21*(4), 307–324. https://doi.org/10.1037/a0037906

4 Schonfeld, I. S., & Bianchi, R. (2016). Burnout and depression: Two entities or one. *Journal of Clinical Psychology, 72*(1), 22–37. https://doi.org/10.1002/jclp.22229

got permission from Wiley to have Renzo as an equal partner in writing the proposal and the book the proposal mapped out.

We don't take for granted that we owe a great deal to modern communication networks. In writing the book, Irvin has mostly worked in Brooklyn, occasionally at the CUNY Graduate Center (kitty-corner from the Empire State Building), Great Neck, New York (less than a mile from the house where Scott Fitzgerald wrote the first chapters of *Gatsby*), and, very occasionally, in Minnesota. Renzo worked in Trondheim, Norway and, from time to time, in Geneva, Switzerland. Although sometimes we communicated via Zoom, we mostly collaborated via email with chunks of text and commentary on the text sailing back and forth day by day, often multiple times in a day. We occasionally had disagreements, which we strove to work out. We take pride in our endeavor because we believe that our work will further the efforts of governments, labor unions, and organizations to protect the health of workers. Workers don't become depressed because there is something in the air. Sometimes elevations in workers' depressive symptoms result from bad job conditions. Our goal is not just to show burnout's overlap with depression and warn against the dangers of its neglect. We also want to underscore the importance of improving working conditions such that job-related depression will be rare and helping workers who have already become depressed to recover.

We organized the book into five chapters. The first provides the reader with a brief (and necessarily partial) history of the very long arc of human knowledge of the condition identified as depression. Within the context of that arc, we show how research has linked depressive conditions to life adversity, including adverse working conditions. The second chapter is devoted to the construct known as burnout, the history of which is millennia shorter than the history of our familiarity with depression. However, from the get-go, burnout has been viewed as a work-related phenomenon and a product of contemporary changes in the economy and the labor market—very much like neurasthenia one century earlier. The third chapter lays out the research on burnout–depression overlap, with an emphasis on our own research efforts. Focusing on burnout–depression overlap allows us to examine the nature of the burnout phenomenon further. The fourth chapter concerns the stigma attached to mental (ill-)health in general, and burnout and depression in particular. The aim of the fifth and final chapter is to show what we can do to help affected workers and prevent more workers from becoming distressed.

We sought to make the book appealing to both professionals (e.g., clinicians, researchers, academics, and graduate students) and educated nonspecialist readers. For the nonspecialists we created two sections, one in Chapter 2 and the other in Chapter 5, that explain in ordinary language some of the technical aspects of the research we review. We also used footnotes at specific junctures in the book to help nonspecialists if that help is needed.

The research we present has excited us. We hope that through this book our sense of excitement carries over to our readers. But ultimately, our foremost desire is that our book be an instrument that helps to make better the lives of people who work.

We thank a number of individuals who helped us with the writing and publication of this book. First, we thank Wiley's Nathanael Mcgavin and Kelly Gomez, who were very helpful in providing us with information we needed in getting our writing done. We thank several individuals who read and made thoughtful editorial suggestions on drafts of different sections of the book when the book was at different stages of completion. These friends, relatives, and colleagues include Romain Brisson, David Kotelchuk, Joel Schwartz, Constance Gemson, Pearl Knopf Schonfeld, Jay Verkuilen, Milton C. Spett, Christina Guthier, and Christian Dormann. Thank you.

1

Occupational Depression

Depression is an important topic. It is a major contributor to the global burden of disease and disability (James et al., 2018). Our goal for the beginning of this chapter is to trace, however briefly, the history of humankind's acquaintance with the disorder. Our forebears have known about depression for millennia. We commonly recognize it in a person when that individual is persistently sad, derives little or no pleasure from the things that ordinarily give pleasure, retreats from getting in touch with friends, and so forth. We will provide a more formal definition of the condition later in the chapter. Although the focal concern of this chapter is work-related depression, by way of an introduction, we briefly address some of the historical background regarding our knowledge of depression in general.

Brief History of Depression

Our brief history commences with the beginning of the recorded word, in Mesopotamia between 2900 and 2300 BCE. The context is *The Epic of Gilgamesh*. King Gilgamesh had been affected by two of life's inevitabilities. First, he is grieving the loss of his friend, Enkidu. The second is his fear of his own eventual death and the fruitless search for a way to avoid it.

Breaking Point: Job Stress, Occupational Depression, and the Myth of Burnout,
First Edition. Irvin Sam Schonfeld and Renzo Bianchi.
© 2025 John Wiley & Sons, Inc. Published 2025 by John Wiley & Sons, Inc.

> Urshanabi said to him, to Gilgamesh:
> "Why are thy cheeks wasted, is sunken [thy face],
> Is so sad thy heart, [are worn thy features]?
> (Why) should there be woe in [thy belly],
> [Thy face be like that] of a wayfarer from afar,
> With cold and heat be seared [thy countenance],
> [As in quest of a wind-puff] thou roamest over the steppe"
> [Gilgamesh] said [to him], to [Urshanabi]: "[Urshanabi, why should my] cheeks
> [not be so wasted], [So sunken my face],
> [So sad] my [heart], so worn my features?
> [(Why) should there not be] woe in [my belly],
> [My face not be like that of a wayfarer from afar],
> Not be so seared [my countenance with cold and heat],
> [And in quest of a wind-puff should I not roam over the steppe]
>
> (Speiser, 1955, p. 91)

We note the sad heart, the somatic symptom of a stomachache, and the dour countenance. Later we will address the difference between depression and mourning, a subject about which Sigmund Freud famously wrote.

Depression, as a human condition, is also evident in several verses in the Hebrew Bible. In Ecclesiastes 1:8, we read: "All things toil to weariness; man cannot utter it, the eye is not satisfied with seeing, nor the ear filled with hearing" (The Jewish Publication Society, 1917). The verse underlines fatigue, anhedonia, and an indifference to life, hallmarks of depression.

Verses 1 and 2 of Psalm 40 are also instructive. The Jewish Publication Society (1917) translates the verses as follows:

1. I waited patiently for the LORD; and He inclined unto me, and heard my cry.
2. He brought me up also out of the tumultuous pit, out of the miry clay; and He set my feet upon a rock, He established my goings.

A more interpretative translation of the verses comes from the Tyndale Bible.

1. I waited patiently for the LORD to help me, and he turned to me and heard my cry.
2. He lifted me out of the pit of despair, out of the mud and the mire.

Tyndale House (1996)

The more interpretative translation refers to King David being in the pit of despair, an indication of his melancholic suffering. We observe despair/sorrow in Psalm 13:3, "How long shall I take counsel in my soul having sorrow in my heart by day?" (The Jewish Publication Society, 1917).

Scattered through the writings of Hippocrates, the Greek physician who lived during the fifth century BCE, is the term "melancholia." In his *Aphorisms*, Hippocrates (1931) described melancholia as "fear and sadness that last a long time." The term is thought to be largely synonymous with depression and is derived from the Greek words for black [μέλαινα] bile [χολή]. Humoralists like Hippocrates and his followers believed that sufferers of depression had an excess of black bile, black bile being one of the four humors, which also include yellow bile, blood, and phlegm. Good health required balance among the humors. Although that belief is considered useless today, Hippocrates and his followers, however, did something of great importance. Hippocrates advanced the idea that physical disorders and melancholia had natural causes (Jackson, 1986). The naturalist hypothesis of Hippocrates was then overlooked for centuries. In the Middle Ages, people commonly believed that some diseases, including melancholia, had supernatural causes, for example, the devil's handiwork or God's punishment (Jackson, 1986).

We observe evidence in Shakespeare's *Hamlet* that Elizabethans understood melancholia.

> ... I have of late—but
> wherefore I know not—lost all my mirth, forgone all
> custom of exercises; and indeed it goes so heavily
> with my disposition that this goodly frame, the
> earth, seems to me a sterile promontory, this most
> excellent canopy, the air, look you, this brave
> o'erhanging firmament, this majestical roof fretted
> with golden fire, why, it appears no other thing to
> me than a foul and pestilent congregation of vapours
> *Thank you, Mr. Jacob Hendon, ISS's*
> *middle school English teacher*

The Hippocratic humoral theory of melancholia, with its idea that an imbalance in bodily humors accompanies melancholy, lived on through the Renaissance. The English scholar Robert Burton, who published *The Anatomy of Melancholy* in 1621, subscribed to a humoral view of depression. The view was commonly held throughout Europe (Sadowsky, 2021).

By the end of the nineteenth century, the mental disorder melancholia was commonly viewed as the province of psychiatry. From the standpoint of clinical science, it is important to reliably distinguish melancholia from other mental disorders. Important milestones in psychiatric classification were achieved in the late nineteenth and early twentieth centuries. In the 1890s, the German psychiatrist Emil Kraepelin developed the beginnings of a nosological system for psychiatry by differentiating manic-depressive psychosis and dementia praecox, which is recognized today as schizophrenia (Jackson, 1986). He used both the symptoms and, based on longitudinal follow-up, the course of the disorder (e.g., whether deteriorating over time or not) to help establish the diagnostic categories. Manic-depressive psychosis included depressed states and manic states (circular insanity), in other words, alterations of depressive and manic periods (today's bipolar disorder). He brought "most melancholic disorders together, eventually to be named manic-depressive insanity" (Jackson, p. 193). As for symptoms of depression, Kraepelin included cognitive slowness, indecisiveness, limiting one's thoughts to life's dark side, exhaustion, and suicidal ideation. Kraepelin was able to discern levels of severity in melancholia from straightforward depression to a depressive condition so severe that it is accompanied by hallucinations and delusions. Kraepelin came to regard these disorders as frequently having a basis in heredity (Jackson, 1986), a far cry from an imbalance involving black bile. He, however, could not pinpoint anatomical markers of these disorders.

In 1904, the Swiss American psychiatrist Adolf Meyer advanced nosology further by distinguishing (unipolar) depression as a category that is separate from Kraepelin's manic-depressive nosological category (Jackson, 1986). Meyer favored the term "depression" over its overripe synonym "melancholia" (Sadowsky, 2021). Meyer tended to regard mental disorder as a pattern of maladaptive responses to the circumstances of life, the patterning depending on "constitution and life experiences" (Jackson, 1986).

What is clear thus far from this brief survey is that from the beginning of recorded time melancholia or depression has been widely observed. But what causes it? As science matured, the idea that the basis for melancholia lies in excessive black bile was recognized as a dead end.

"Depression is rage turned inward," Dr. Jennifer Melfi

Beginning in the late 1890s and continuing onward into the next century, the psychoanalytic movement had much to say about mental disorders, including depression, and came to dominate psychiatry for much of the twentieth century. The German psychoanalyst Karl Abraham (1968/1911) observed the similarities of grief or sadness, on one hand, and depression, on the other. He then suggested an important difference. Abraham advanced the view that depression is unconsciously motivated.

Sigmund Freud (1953–1974/1917) graciously allowed Abraham's observation to be the point of departure for the influential paper "Mourning and Melancholia," although Freud had made the grief–depression comparison even earlier than Abraham.[1] In "Mourning and Melancholia," Freud wrote that "although mourning involves grave departures from the normal attitude to life, it never occurs to us to regard it as a pathological condition" (p. 243). The mental features of melancholia include "a profoundly painful dejection, cessation of interest in the outside world, loss of the capacity to love, inhibition of all activity, and a lowering of the self-regarding feelings to a degree that finds utterance in self-reproaches" (p. 244). Freud noted that individuals who mourn a person they loved share many of the same features as the melancholic, but with one notable exception, namely, disturbed self-regard.

Freud observed that in mourning, eventually the individual who suffered a loss, as grief-stricken as the individual is at first, gradually comes to regain an interest in the world. He called that transition "the work of mourning." The person suffering from melancholia may have, indeed, suffered a loss of varying degrees of personal importance, ranging from

---

1 Noted by James Strachey, the editor of *The Standard Edition of the Complete Psychological Works of Sigmund Freud*.

the death of a parent with whom the melancholic has had an ambivalent relationship to a romantic relationship that ended when one partner jilted the other to a personal slight from a close friend. In melancholia, Freud pointed out that the degree of symptom manifestation and duration is greatly out of proportion to the magnitude of the loss. In Freud's estimation, melancholics regard themselves as "worthless, incapable of any achievement and morally despicable."

Freud outlined what he regarded as a major cause of depression by attempting to solve the riddle of that surmised disproportion. He wrote, "If one listens patiently to a melancholic's many and various self-accusations, one cannot in the end avoid the impression that often the most violent of them are hardly at all applicable to the patient himself, but that with insignificant modifications they do fit someone else, someone whom the patient loves or has loved or should love" (p. 248). Freud viewed the self-reproaches of melancholics as reproaches against a love object that have been unconsciously displaced onto the self. To reproach another who is (or should be) much loved (e.g., a mother or a father) is impermissible. Murderous rage against a love object gets displaced, becoming suicidal ideation. The treatment for melancholia is then psychoanalysis, an important goal of which is to make what has been unconscious conscious.

The quotation (Figgis et al., 2004) that heads this section comes from an episode of a popular TV crime series about a mobster named Tony Soprano who operates in northern New Jersey. Unknown to the soldiers and capos in Tony's crime family and the crime families of his rivals, he sees a psychiatrist named Jennifer Melfi for treatment of his mental health problems. The episode we quoted was first broadcast in 2004, more than 87 years after the publication—in German—of *Mourning and Melancholia* and continues to be broadcast, evidence of the staying power of Freud's ideas regarding a principal cause of depression.

Challenge to Freud's Explanation of Depression

Freud's theory of depression and other mental disorders (e.g., schizophrenia) has not been without critics. The Austrian British philosopher of science Karl Popper (1963) advanced the view that psychoanalytic theory should not even be regarded as a scientific theory. Popper rejected the tendency of adherents of psychoanalysis to interpret many kinds of human interactions as evidence for the truth of psychoanalytic theory. The first author, to help undergraduates attending his research course, created an illustrative example of what Popper meant. Here is an excerpt from that course.

> A psychoanalyst would find consistent with psychoanalytic theory the following observations. A pair of overprotecting parents living in the Park Slope section of Brooklyn raises a very hostile boy. The analyst asserts that the parents' overprotectiveness unconsciously generates belligerence in the offspring, who directs hostility to other neighborhood children, suspecting that they "are out to get him." Another pair of overprotecting parents from the same neighborhood has a nervous boy. The analyst claims that the parents unconsciously and excessively communicate to the child that the other children in the neighborhood are dangerous delinquents, causing the boy to be meek and avoidant. Yet another pair overprotecting parents living in the same neighborhood has a normal boy and somehow that gets explained by the analyst. The psychoanalyst can somehow explain what takes place in every kind of parent–child constellation.

There was more to the classroom discussion of Popper's views, but the foregoing example provides a flavor for what Popper thought of psychoanalytic theory. It explains everything, but it explains everything post hoc. Professionals allied to the psychoanalytic movement have failed to make predictions (hypotheses) in advance of collecting observations. By making such advance predictions, then collecting observations, these professionals could test the truth value of the predictions. Popper (1963) underlined the idea that it is important for science that scientific theories be able to generate hypotheses that are falsifiable. By that he meant that scientists need to show that theories generate hypotheses that can be shown, in principle, to be incompatible with the observations collected in a research endeavor. In plain English, the scientist proposing a hypothesis "goes out on a limb." The scientist collects data that can be consistent with the hypothesis or contradict the hypothesis. Theories that generate hypotheses that are demonstrated to be consistent with the collected observations gain status in the scientific community. Theories that generate hypotheses that are inconsistent with observations lose status. The problem with psychoanalytic theory, according to Popper, is that it fails to generate falsifiable, that is, testable, hypotheses at all (in Chapter 3 we return to Popper's ideas regarding hypothesis-testing, but in a different context). The American psychiatrist Aaron Beck was to our knowledge the first researcher to put psychoanalytic theory to the test.

Aaron Beck and Albert Ellis trained to become and indeed became practitioners of psychoanalysis. They both, however, evolved into apostates, rejecting psychoanalytic theories. Both men independently went on to develop cognitive therapies that contrast with psychoanalysis. Their therapies were nonetheless designed to help individuals with depression and other mental health problems. Ellis (1958), an American psychologist, broke away from psychoanalysis first. He viewed maladaptive behavior patterns as the result of irrational thinking and beliefs that have been learned. He developed a psychotherapy called rational therapy that later evolved into rational emotive therapy and that further evolved into rational emotive behavior therapy. Ellis's approach to psychotherapy employs something like a Socratic dialogue and disputation to help individuals discover what is false or misleading in their thinking, correct that thinking, and thereby get clients to lead happier, more productive lives. Ellis's approach influenced later cognitively oriented therapies for depression and other mental health problems (see Chapter 5).

Like Ellis, Beck was a psychotherapist. Beck, however, differed from Ellis in an important way. Beck was also a researcher. He and his colleague Marvin Hurvich (1959) conducted a study in which the dreams of depressed and nondepressed patients were transcribed and evaluated by two raters. The authors hypothesized that, compared to the dreams of the nondepressed, the dreams of depressed patients would be characterized by disappointment, sorrow, loneliness, and rejection. Beck also conducted a follow-up study with a larger sample, again finding similar results (Beck & Ward, 1961). But Beck and his colleagues made an easy prediction, namely, that, compared to the nondepressed, depressed individuals would report more depressive features in their dreams. The dreams in the depressed samples were consistent with what depressed individuals experience in their waking thoughts and feelings.

The test of psychoanalytic theory should be more nuanced. To understand that nuance, we should turn to the theory's axioms bearing on dreams.

If we restrict ourselves to the minimum of new knowledge which has been established with certainty, we can still say this of dreams: they have proved that *what is suppressed continues to exist in normal people as well as abnormal, and remains capable of psychical functioning* [italics by the authors]. Dreams themselves are among the manifestations of this suppressed material.... (Freud, 1953–1974/1899, p. 608).

According to Freudian theory, during waking life an unconscious mental censor protects against id-related unconscious content, such as unacceptable sexual and aggressive thoughts and feelings, entering a person's consciousness. During sleep, however, the censor relaxes somewhat, allowing the unacceptable content to emerge, slightly disguised by "dream work," and that content plays a part in dreams. If dreams are the king's highway to the unconscious, then dreams should, consistent with psychoanalytic theory, reveal content that underscores anger or hostility directed at a loved one or another important figure in a person's life. An expression of that anger would ordinarily be deemed unacceptable in everyday family and social life. A Popperian hypothesis that would follow from psychoanalytic theory would be that, compared to the dreams of the nondepressed, the dreams of depressed individuals would show more other-directed angry and hostile imagery, which was not what Beck found.

Beck (personal communication to ISS, 2014) reported that he and his colleague Hurvich unexpectedly found *less* evidence of hostile content in the dreams of the depressed patients than in the dreams of the nondepressed patients, contradicting the abovementioned Popperian hypothesis that would follow from psychoanalytic theory, a hypothesis they did not include in their 1959 and, for that matter, Beck and Ward's 1961 paper. The papers were published before Beck's transition away from psychoanalytic orthodoxy. Beck's research and clinical observations led to his break with psychoanalytic orthodoxy. Beck went on to develop a cognitively oriented therapy designed to help individuals suffering from depression (Beck, 2019), a therapy we describe in Chapter 5.

Helplessness and Hopelessness

The purpose of the learned helplessness theory of depression, developed by psychologist Martin E. Seligman and behavioral neuroscientist Steven F. Maier, was to explain how individuals may come to regard themselves as powerless and become passive in the face of adversity (for reviews, see Seligman, 1975, and Peterson et al., 1993). The theory emerged from a series of experiments conducted in the 1960s (e.g., Overmier & Seligman, 1967; Seligman & Maier, 1967). The experiments showed that dogs that experienced uncontrollable and inescapable electric shocks did not attempt to escape even when given the opportunity to do so. They had learned to be helpless.

Seligman and Maier extrapolated these findings, suggesting that similar processes could occur in humans. According to their theory, when individuals repeatedly face negative situations that they perceive as beyond their control, they may learn that they have no agency over their environment. This belief in the inability to change or influence outcomes can lead to a state of passivity and depression.

The learned helplessness theory emphasizes the importance of three factors:

- Contingency: the perceived lack of relationship between one's behavior and the outcome of events.
- Cognition: the development of a belief that outcomes are uncontrollable.
- Behavior: a resulting passive or depressive response due to the belief that one cannot influence outcomes.

Learned helplessness theory has been influential in understanding cognitive aspects of depression, underlining how beliefs about control and efficacy can influence health (e.g., De Raedt & Hooley, 2016; Grahek et al., 2019; Moscarello & Hartley, 2017). The theory led to further research into cognitive-behavioral mechanisms and therapies designed to counteract these learned beliefs by fostering a sense of control and efficacy in individuals.

The original learned helplessness theory underwent significant refinement over the years, leading to a more nuanced understanding of how learned helplessness relates to depression and other psychological conditions (e.g., anxiety). Key developments in this evolution included an "attributional reformulation" (Abramson et al., 1978). Building on the initial theory, so-called *attributional styles* were introduced as an important factor in the learned helplessness model. This reformulation proposed that the way individuals explain the causes of negative events—whether they assess these causes as internal or external to themselves, stable or unstable, and global (pan-situational) or situation specific—influences their likelihood of developing learned helplessness. People who habitually interpret setbacks as permanent, pervasive, and due to personal failings are more likely to become depressed.

Abramson et al. (1989) revised the attributional reformulation of the theory, introducing the *hopelessness theory of depression*: "According to the hopelessness theory, a proximal sufficient cause of the symptoms of hopelessness depression is an expectation that highly desired outcomes will not occur or that highly aversive outcomes will occur coupled with an expectation that no response in one's repertoire will change the likelihood of occurrence of these outcomes" (p. 359). Hopelessness theory refined the learned helplessness model, notably by offering a more detailed framework for understanding how cognitive factors contribute to the development of depression, emphasizing the role of pessimistic expectations about the future (Alloy et al., 2006; Liu et al., 2015). We connect to this attributional reformulation in Chapter 3 when we explore how burnout connects to a depressive cognitive style.

Early Linkages of Work to Psychological State

The Italian physician Bernardino Ramazzini (1700/1750), the father of occupational medicine, is perhaps the first person to systematically link work to disease. The first edition of his magnum opus was published in Latin as *De Morbis Artificum Diatriba* [Diseases of Workers] in 1700 and translated into English in 1750. He may have been the first writer to link specific occupations to specific illnesses. For example, he understood something about musculoskeletal disorders. He found that clerks, because of their constant sitting and bookkeeping activities, experience a great deal of fatigue including fatigue of the arm. Ramazzini found that sedentary workers are subject to lumbago. He also found that melancholia plagues scholars. He wrote, "we find, that studious Persons, though naturally of jovial merry Temper, do, in Process of Time, become melancholy and heavy" (p. 271). Ramazzini also found that stomachaches are prevalent in men of learning "because the animal spirits are diverted, and taken up in the intellectual Service; or these Spirits are not conveyed to the Stomach with sufficient Influx" (p. 270). "Animal spirits" were thought to be important to the smooth running of the viscera but cause problems when they are diverted to the brain. He also suggested that fatigue falls heavily on scholars.

The Scottish philosopher and economist Adam Smith makes a surprise visit to these pages. He was the author of *An Inquiry into the Nature and Causes of the Wealth of Nations*, which is also known by its shorter title *The Wealth of Nations*, a text that builds a case for a laissez-faire economy, free markets, and the division of labor. Published in 1776, at the dawn of the Industrial Revolution, Smith describes a pin factory in two different circumstances. In one, each worker in the factory builds an entire pin from scratch. In the other circumstance, wealth-building economies of scale are obtained with a division of labor. In that latter case one worker repeatedly makes one facet of the pin (e.g., "draws out the wire") and passes the work to the next worker, who performs the next facet of pin-making (e.g., straightens the wire), and so on until a final worker places the head on the pin. Smith describes 18 distinct operations. Each worker repeats over and over the operation with which the worker was tasked.

Smith understood that having workers repetitively engage in simple tasks all day would have a deleterious effect on the workers' psychological functioning (Schonfeld & Chang, 2017). He wrote that the laborer "generally becomes as stupid and ignorant as it is possible for a human creature. The torpor of his mind renders him, not only incapable of relishing or bearing a part in any rational conversation, but of conceiving any generous, noble, or tender sentiment" (p. 303, Vol. 2). While Smith did not use the term "melancholia," the mental torpor of mind to which he referred is either melancholia or a condition that is adjacent to melancholia. Although Smith was generally opposed to governments interfering with the economy (except in the case of government regulation of banks), he wrote that this is the fate of "the laboring poor, that is, the great body of the people ... unless government takes some pains to prevent it" (p. 303, Vol. 2).

Not surprisingly, we turn to Smith's antithesis, Karl Marx. He was concerned with the impact of industrialization on the industrial worker.

Marx (1967/1844) advanced the concept of alienation, which has important implications for psychology. The concept has several different but related senses. In one sense, alienation refers to industrial workers losing the ability to direct their own lives, including their labor. In another sense, alienation can mean that a worker can feel estranged from fellow workers and other human beings. A worker has become a commodity, an easily replaceable and salable part of a giant industrial flywheel. In yet another sense of the term "alienation," industrial workers, unlike the artisans they replaced, are distanced from the goods they create.

Marx, like Smith, underscored the psychological impact of the brutalization of the division of labor in industrial production. Work, Marx noted, is drained of intrinsic satisfaction. With increasing exertion, monotony, and repetitiveness, "the poorer [the worker] and his inner world become." Although neither Marx nor Smith used the term "melancholia," we find an echo of that concept in their writing about the psychological impact of industrialization and the division of labor on the worker.

In his book *The Division of Labor in Society*, Émile Durkheim (1984/1893), the French sociologist, underlined the benefits of the division of labor. For example, the division of labor, he argued, creates mutual dependency and social integration. He also observed that industries, because they expand markets beyond local areas, can become national or even international in scope. He wrote that because consumers are dispersed, the producer "can no longer figure out to himself [the market's] limits" with production lacking "any check or regulation," which can lead to miscalculations—upward or downward—of the size of demand (p. 305). This condition results in "crises that periodically disturb economic functions" (p. 305). Durkheim called the lack of regulation in the economy "anomie." He argued against unfettered capitalism and supported the idea of government regulation of the economy to mitigate the deleterious effects of wild swings in the economy.

The idea of anomie has implications for human psychology. Durkheim (1951/1912) later connected anomie to the risk of suicide. Using official data collected in several European countries, he found that the number of suicides increases during both downward *and* upward swings in the business cycle. He advanced the view that poverty per se does not increase the rate of suicide.

> If therefore industrial or financial crises increase suicides, this is not because they cause poverty, since crises of prosperity have the same result; it is because they are crises, that is, disturbances of the collective order. Every disturbance of equilibrium, even though it achieves greater comfort and a heightening of general vitality, is an impulse to voluntary death. (p. 246)

Psychiatry has long linked suicidal ideation, attempted suicide, and completed suicide to depression. What, according to Durkheim, is occurring at the level of the individual that leads to suicide? In Durkheim's view, individuals who have attained wealth may develop an "inextinguishable thirst" for more and more pleasures and drive themselves into a "state of perpetual unhappiness." By contrast, "[i]n the case of economic disasters," something else comes into play, according to Durkheim. Life has dramatically changed. The individual experiences a need to repress wants and engage in an unaccustomed level of self-control. This "reduced existence" is intolerable.

The experience of modern industrial workers is important to look at. The Ford assembly line could be a case study. With the refinement of the assembly line at Ford plants in Michigan, an underside emerged, namely, that of the "increasing dehumanization of workers" (Wallace, 2003). Wallace described the plants as run like a "totalitarian state in miniature." There was even an organization in the plant, one with the anodyne name of "Service Department," that line workers nicknamed "Ford's Gestapo." It was staffed by ex-convicts, former prizefighters, and informants. Workers who aroused suspicions that they were unhappy with Ford were beaten by Service Department thugs. Ford workers despised, and feared, the Service Department (Cruden, 1932). The fast-paced assembly line allowed for little time for rest or toilet breaks (Linder & Nygaard, 1998). Ford concealed the true accident rates at its plants by sending accident victims to Ford's own hospital (Cruden, 1932). Many men at the plant suspected, although an understandable exaggeration, that one man per day was killed in an industrial accident; on one of the days that Cruden worked, six men were accidentally killed—deaths at the plant would be difficult to conceal. Cruden reported that feelings of cynicism, discontent, and distress were prevalent among Ford's factory workers. During the Great Depression, many Ford workers were trapped in their jobs because alternative work was difficult to obtain.

Part of the impact of work also involves the experience of involuntary unemployment. In 1933, Marie Jahoda, one of the first women to attain renown in the male-dominated social sciences, published, along with her husband Paul F. Lazarsfeld and their colleague Hans Zeisel, a trailblazing book entitled *Marienthal: The Sociography of an Unemployed Community* (1971/1933). The book detailed their research on the residents of a small Austrian community in which *all* adults were unemployed throughout the late 1920s and early 1930s.

Jahoda et al. found that over time community members became less and less engaged in everyday activities. The research team documented the community members' growing apathy. Between 1929 and 1931, on average the number of books residents borrowed from the town library decreased. Local membership in the leading political party declined. Life history interviews with residents revealed an aimlessness in their lives. An observer may see "heartrending outbursts of despair." The team detailed "the paralyzing effects of unemployment." Thus, Jahoda and her colleagues documented the psychological costs of involuntary unemployment, which, taking place during the Great Depression, had the look and feel of psychological depression.

The Diagnosis of Depression

To pave the way for our look at research bearing on the relation of work to depression, we consider two ways in which depression has been thought of. We begin with one of those two ways, a diagnosis. According to modern psychiatry's most favored definition of depression, which is found in the *Diagnostic and Statistical Manual* (*DSM–5*) of the American Psychiatric Association (APA, 2013) and its most recent revision (APA, 2022), to be diagnosed with major depressive disorder (MDD),[2] individuals must meet several symptom criteria. First, they must experience at least one of two symptoms nearly every day for almost two consecutive weeks. The two required symptoms are either anhedonia or depressed mood. Anhedonia refers to a person being unable to experience

---

2 MDD is also called major depression, clinical depression, or a major depressive episode.

pleasure in everyday life—a nice cup of coffee or a walk in the park. We are not describing sexual pleasure, just the ordinary, everyday variety of pleasure that people normally enjoy. The other required symptom, depressed mood, refers to feelings of dejection, hopelessness, and/or sadness. The cloak of sadness occurs even without having suffered the loss of a loved one.

In addition, to meet the criteria for a diagnosis of MDD, an individual must show evidence of experiencing at least four of seven other symptoms. If the individual shows evidence of both anhedonia and depressed mood, the person needs to manifest at least three of the other seven symptoms to meet the criteria for a diagnosis.

These seven other symptoms include change in appetite, disturbed sleep, psychomotor alterations, fatigue, feelings of worthlessness, cognitive impairment, and thoughts of death. Except for thoughts of death, the other symptoms must be experienced almost every day over the same two-week period anhedonia and/or depressed mood are experienced.

Change in appetite refers to a dietary change that leads to dramatic weight loss or gain. Disturbed sleep refers to difficulty falling or staying asleep (insomnia). Disturbed sleep could also refer to sleeping way too much (hypersomnia). Psychomotor alterations include psychomotor agitation, restlessness, or fidgeting. They could also reflect the opposite, in which the affected individual moves unusually slowly (psychomotor retardation). The fatigue symptom involves the loss of energy or feeling tired much of the time. Feelings of worthlessness include feeling like a failure, having let down members of one's family, or experiencing excessive and inappropriate guilt. Cognitive impairment refers to the individual experiencing difficulties thinking, concentrating, or paying attention. The individual may also be unusually indecisive.

The seventh symptom involves "recurrent thoughts of death" (APA, 2013). These thoughts can reflect the affected person's idea of being better off if no longer alive. Individuals are considered positive for this symptom regardless of having a specific plan to end their lives or attempt suicide. This last symptom counts toward a diagnosis of MDD even if it is experienced for a day or two during the two-week period. The symptom is too important to ignore.

There is one additional criterion for a diagnosis. The symptoms must have caused "clinically significant distress or impairment in social, occupational, or other important areas of functioning" (APA, 2013).

Finally, the pattern of symptoms cannot be attributed to the effects of substance use or a medical condition. The *DSM-5*'s approach to diagnosing major depression comports with the diagnostic criteria in the latest edition of the *International Classification of Diseases* (https://icd.who.int/browse/2024-01/mms/en#1563440232; World Health Organization, 2024).

A diagnosis of depression or any other mental disorder is made by way of a clinical interview. Sometimes a person close to the individual could provide background information to the clinician. The *DSM-5* observes that "[o]ften insomnia or fatigue is the presenting complaint, and a failure to probe for accompanying depressive symptoms will result in underdiagnosis" (p. 162). Although not part of the diagnosis, other symptoms, including anxiety, complaints about physical health, irritability, and tearfulness, often co-occur with depression (American Psychiatric Association, 2013; World Health Organization, 2024). Depression is also associated with higher risk of mortality from illness or accident. A diagnosis can be further refined using specifiers, for example, major depressive disorder with atypical features. The latter specifier "atypical" does not refer to a low prevalence. Rather it means that among these depressed individuals, several other patterns emerge including a mood that can occasionally brighten, a significant increase in appetite or weight, hypersomnia, a sensitivity to interpersonal rejection that impairs social relations, and leaden feelings in the limbs.

Another Way to Think About Depression

The philosopher of science Carl Hempel (1961) noted that in the sciences categorical classification often gives way to a dimensional approach to phenomena. Besides the diagnostic conceptualization of depression, there is another way to conceptualize it, a dimensional way. Instead of regarding depression as an entity that is either present or absent, one can also conceptualize depression as a continuum, like temperature. To meet criteria for a diagnosis, an individual must manifest at least five symptoms for specified durations. But what about an individual who manifests fewer than the five symptoms or experiences those symptoms but less often than nearly every day during a two-week period? That individual does not meet criteria for a diagnosis. Nevertheless, something is going

CONTINUUM OF DEPRESSION

```
                                            Clinical stage
┌─────────────────────────────────────────┐
│  INCREASING SYMPTOM INTENSITY/FREQUENCY │──▶
└─────────────────────────────────────────┘
Low end of the                        High end of the
continuum                             continuum
```

Figure 1.1 The relation of depression as a continuum to depression as a diagnosis.

wrong for the individual. But what? If we think of depression as a continuum, we have a better idea of the "what."

Using a general population sample, Dohrenwend et al. (1980) found that several psychological symptom scales were "strongly intercorrelated relative to their reliabilities."[3] These scales assessed such symptoms as dread, sadness, hopelessness, poor self-esteem, guilt, enervation, confused thinking (e.g., trouble concentrating), and anxiety. Moreover, the symptoms each scale assesses are, except for anxiety, markers of depression. Anxiety, however, is part of that underlying dimension and is a condition that is associated with depression (APA, 2013). Later studies at the frontiers of research on psychopathology have provided evidence that depression *can* be conceptualized as a continuum (Haslam et al., 2012; Kotov et al., 2017; Liu, 2016; Pickles & Angold, 2003). The research, moreover, suggests that depression and anxiety are part of the same continuum of internalizing psychopathology[4] (Schonfeld et al., 2019). Individuals who manifest very high scores on psychological symptom scales that reflect that continuum are likely to meet criteria for a diagnosis of MDD. But people with intermediate positions on the continuum also suffer their own commensurate measure of psychological distress.[5] Figure 1.1 illustrates the relation between depression as a continuous factor and depression as a clinical diagnosis.

---

[3] The reliability mentioned here reflects the extent to which the kernel of a scale, as opposed to the measurement error a scale score also carries, reflects something dependable. A scale's reliability coefficient sets an upper limit on a correlation coefficient. See Chapter 2 for further discussion of reliability.

[4] There is also an externalizing dimension of psychopathology that includes aggressive behavior, risky sexual behavior, and so forth (Haslam et al., 2012).

[5] Some authors regard MDD and depressive symptoms measured as a continuous factor to be different entities (Kendler & Aggen, 2023).

Assessing Depression in the Research Context

We have established that researchers treat depression in either of two ways. The first is that of a diagnosis that is present or absent. A diagnosis is ascertained in a research context with the help of a clinical interview, often a structured interview with some limited ways for the interviewer to diverge from the interview text when a research participant's answers are unclear. Several semistructured diagnostic interviews are available for research purposes; three of the most prominent are the Schedule of Affective Disorders and Schizophrenia or SADS (Endicott & Spitzer, 1978; Fawcett, 2013); the Structured Clinical Interview for *DSM–III* or SCID (Riskind et al., 1987), and the Composite International Diagnostic Interview or CIDI (World Health Organization, 1990). We also underline that the interviews have been subject to revisions over time or have variants that address current disorders or disorders that have occurred over a lifetime.

The second way to treat depression is as a continuous dimension. In this case, the number of assessment instruments grows. We can employ psychological symptom scales that can be completed either as interviews or questionnaires. Among these is an alphabet soup of assessment instruments including the BDI, CES-D, DASS, GHQ, HADS, HRSD, HSCL, MMPI-D, ODI, PHQ-9, POMS, SCL-90-R, and so forth. Each assesses depression on a continuum either as a stand-alone scale (like the PHQ-9) or as part of a package that includes one or more other psychological symptom scales (like the DASS). Researchers have conducted psychometric research to validate each scale. Validating a scale refers to adducing evidence sufficient to show that the scale measures the target construct, in this case depression as a continuous factor. Although clinical interviews have been used in research on the impact of adverse working conditions, depressive symptom scales have been employed more often in such research.

"The Stress of Life"

Research on life stress has provided a foundation for research on the social origins of depression. Building on research conducted by Walter B. Cannon 30 and 40 years earlier, Hans Selye, in 1956, published a book entitled *The Stress of Life* and published a revised edition in 1976. Selye's research, which was concerned with how an organism responds physiologically to environmental stimuli, particularly stimuli most of us would term "stressful," had implications for depression research to come. He pioneered research on the hypothalamic–pituitary–adrenal (HPA), or stress, axis (see Schonfeld & Chang, 2017). Although Selye was not specifically interested in job-related stress, his research, nonetheless, influenced investigators who were interested in studying job stress.

In 1957, Norman G. Hawkins, Roberts Davies, and Thomas H. Holmes, in a paper they published in a tuberculosis and pulmonary disease journal, noted that "[f]or twenty-five hundred years or more some physicians have believed that tuberculosis was frequently initiated by unhappy or stressful experiences" (p. 768). In 1964, Richard H. Rahe, Holmes, and their colleagues published a paper in which they carried out research that employed Hawkins et al.'s measure of social stressors. Although not a flawless study from a methodological standpoint (e.g., recall bias), Rahe and colleagues found that social stressors preceded the diagnosis of tuberculosis, cardiac disease, dermatologic disease, and inguinal hernia and antedated unwed pregnancies.

Several methodologically stronger studies (Friedman et al., 1958; Kasl & Cobb, 1970; Levi, 1972; Cobb & Rose, 1973) demonstrated that we can investigate the impact of job stressors on health. Meyer Friedman, Ray Rosenman, and Vernice Carroll found that, independent of risk factors such as diet and exercise, severe job stress in the form of highly excessive workloads adversely affected serum cholesterol levels and blood clotting time in male accountants. Stanislav Kasl and Sydney Cobb linked involuntary unemployment in male factory workers to elevations in blood pressure. Lennart Levi showed that a change from hourly wages to piecework was followed by increases in adrenaline and noradrenaline in women invoicing clerks; a reversion to hourly wages was attended by a decline. In another all-male sample, Sydney Cobb and Robert Rose linked the intensity of air traffic to hypertension and peptic ulcer in air traffic controllers.

A challenge that emerged was to show that methodologically strong research could demonstrate a link between working conditions and psychological symptoms. Katharine Parkes (1982) met that challenge.

Capitalizing on a natural experiment, Parkes showed that compared to rotations into surgical wards, when student nurses rotated into medical wards, which put "greater affective demands" on them, they manifested higher levels of depressive symptoms.

Perhaps the first person to use a phrase that is a variant of the term "occupational depression" was Maureen Oswin (1978). Oswin, a British nurse, identified a phenomenon she called "professional depression." Although these were uncontrolled, qualitative observations, Oswin convincingly linked professional depression to adverse working conditions at an understaffed, long-term-care hospital that served severely handicapped children. She reported on working conditions that included a lack of support from the hospital administration, meals arriving late from the central kitchen, crises during feeding, and having to deal with children who were difficult to feed. The work was complicated by a continuing shortage of nurses that was sustained by the stressfulness of the job. Many years later, the authors of this book developed a measure of occupational depression entitled the Occupational Depression Inventory (ODI; Bianchi & Schonfeld, 2020; Schonfeld & Bianchi, 2022). The ODI is described in some detail in Chapter 3 and is included in the Appendix.

Stressful Life Events

The foundation of research on stressful job conditions, conditions that could potentially lead to clinical depression or elevations in depressive symptoms, derives from research aimed at identifying the stressful conditions of life in general. The year 1967 is a reasonably good starting point for this disquisition. During that year, Thomas H. Holmes and Richard H. Rahe, both psychiatrists, built on their earlier work (Rahe et al., 1964) and published a paper describing their new Social Readjustment Rating Scale (SRRS). The SRRS could be administered by interview or questionnaire. Researchers can use the instrument to ascertain whether an individual experienced any of 43 life events. The events were derived from clinical experience and reflect the influence of Adolf Meyer on Holmes and Rahe. Meyer advanced the goal of helping psychiatrists better understand an individual's life circumstances. The events on the SRRS included marriage, vacation, divorce, getting fired, death of a loved one, and so forth and how much of a life adjustment an individual would, on average, make upon experiencing the event. Aside from estimating how much readjustment each event requires, some of the events in question are ordinarily positive and others, stressful.

The paper by Holmes and Rahe proved to be influential. In 2006, Bruce P. Dohrenwend wrote that following the publication of their SRRS, "a tremendous increase has occurred in the construction of such measures and in quantitative research on relations between inventoried life events and health" (p. 477). By January 2024, the paper was cited more than 7,700 times.

Influenced by Holmes and Rahe, other investigators began to create measures to assess stressful life events (SLEs). Some of those investigators examined SLEs' link to depression, as a diagnosis. Others examined SLEs' link to depressive symptoms, as assessed by psychological symptom scales. For example, Barbara Snell Dohrenwend (1973) linked SLEs to a composite measure of psychosomatic, anxiety, and depressive symptoms. She also linked the risk of exposure to SLEs to lower social statuses.

George W. Brown and Tirril Harris (1978), in their groundbreaking book, *The Social Origins of Depression*, concerned themselves with social factors that increase the risk of clinical depression, as diagnosed by clinical interview. In a study of women who lived in the Camberwell borough of London, Brown and Harris examined the link between depression and SLEs, but only SLEs that likely occurred independently of the women's personalities. An example of such an event is the woman's husband getting unexpectedly laid off. The question of SLE independence was important because the authors were concerned about the confounding of event, personality, and mental disorder. They excluded events that a research participant, by virtue of her personality, could arguably have contributed to.

Brown and Harris also extended the concept of SLEs to the idea of "difficulties," which represented disagreeable conditions that lasted four or more weeks (e.g., a damp apartment or a son who uses illicit drugs). They, surprisingly, did not find that SLEs or difficulties alone predicted clinical depression. The authors, however, did find that an SLE or difficulty occurring in combination with what they termed a "vulnerability factor" increased the risk of depression. An example of a vulnerability factor[6] is the absence of a *confidant*, that is, another person—a husband or a friend—with whom the woman had a close and confiding relationship, someone in whom the woman could tell anything about herself without feeling embarrassed. Another vulnerability is lower social class with its attendant woes, such as meager income or substandard housing. Interestingly, the vulnerability factors on their own did not lead to an episode of depression; however, they served as the ground on which an SLE or difficulty landed, and the combination of an SLE or difficulty with a vulnerability increased the risk of clinical depression.

An SLE and a vulnerability factor can be termed risk factors, in this case risk factors for depression. The risk factors had a combined impact on depression that was different from—in this case greater than—the sum of the singular impacts of each factor. In research parlance, a combined effect of the impact of which is greater than the sum of the individual effects of each factor—a kind of synergy of misfortune—represents an interaction. The idea of an interaction also emerges in the demand-control model of the impact of working conditions on the health of workers, a model we discuss later in this chapter.

In addition to studies linking SLEs to depression as a diagnosis, other research that grew out of Holmes and Rahe's initial work linked SLEs to elevations in depressive symptoms. For example, Monroe et al. (1986), in a study of married Pennsylvania women having low depressive symptom levels at baseline, found that SLEs and reduced social support at baseline predicted depressive symptoms one year later. Importantly, the investigators statistically controlled for baseline

---

6 Brown, a sociologist, and Harris, a psychoanalytically oriented psychotherapist, also included among the vulnerability factors, early loss of a woman's mother. Given their combined interest in Freud, John Bowlby, and Aaron Beck, they developed a theory about the impact of an SLE on a woman who had suffered maternal loss at age 11 or younger, the psychological residua of that loss creating a base with which the adult experience of an SLE would resonate to provoke an episode of depression. They, however, revised their theory given later evidence they collected. In a study of the impact of SLEs in women who experienced early maternal loss (through death or separation), they (Harris et al., 1986) found that if the quality of care following the loss (e.g., the father pulled himself together to take good care of his daughter), the woman was no more vulnerable to a depressive episode following an SLE than a woman who did not experience such a loss and but later was subject to an SLE. Harris et al. found that inadequacy of care following early maternal loss is the vulnerability factor, not the loss per se.

symptoms in view of the potential for any confounding of the reporting of SLEs and symptoms.

Studies of general life stress have provided a backdrop for research on the relation of working conditions to heightened depressive symptom levels. Working conditions can be episodic like SLEs. Or they can be ongoing, like Brown and Harris's (1978) difficulties. Individuals exposed to episodic or ongoing stressors at work, just as individuals exposed to such stressors outside of work, can be put at risk.

An example of Holmes and Rahe's influence (by way of Dohrenwend [1979; Dohrenwend et al., 1987]) on research on working conditions comes from Schonfeld's (2001) study of job stressors affecting women who were first-year New York City public school teachers.[7] For SLEs, Schonfeld assessed the frequencies of episodically occurring classroom stressors (e.g., a fight between students, a student threatening the teacher). He also assessed ongoing stressors (e.g., an overcrowded classroom, a vandalized classroom going unrepaired) loosely paralleling Brown and Harris's (1978) concept of difficulties. Schonfeld mixed a few positively worded items (e.g., praise from an administrator) among the stressor questions to reduce the risk of "response sets"[8] and ensure that the teachers paid careful attention.

Because official reports of stressful school conditions have been defective (e.g., violence against teachers being woefully underreported; Bloch, 1978; Schonfeld, 1992), Schonfeld designed special self-report stressor measures instead of relying on official records. These measures were "neutral self-reports," a just-the-facts type of measure (Kasl, 1987). In many earlier studies, researchers had respondents inject their feelings into stressor frequency measures, creating an artifact that likely increased the magnitude of the correlation between the stressor scales

---

7 The first author was for six years a mathematics teacher in a New York City public school. During that period, he did not anticipate that one day he would conduct research on the impact of job stress on teachers. His psychology-related research interests at the time he was a teacher lay in cognitive development as he pursued a master's degree in night school. But during that period, he became aware of the considerable burden of job stress affecting many teachers in his school. The stress came in the form of assaults, threats of assault, and generally discourteous student behavior.

8 A response set is a tendency for a research participant to respond to scale items in an excessively consistent way, such as a tendency to respond to items about the occurrence of episodic events "Not at all" or "Once per week," no matter the actual frequency of the events identified in the items.

and psychological symptoms. Concerned that teacher distress could still bias the reporting of job stressors (e.g., a distressed teacher overreporting student misbehavior), Schonfeld (1996, 2001) found that the neutrally worded stressor reports obtained during the fall and spring terms were minimally confounded with depressive symptoms he assessed during the summer pre-employment period.

Consistent with his hypothesis bearing on the importance of control in the work environment, Schonfeld (2001) found that increasing exposure to episodic and ongoing stressors predicted immediate and later elevations in depressive symptoms, with no evidence of reverse causation.[9] Schonfeld also found that the supportiveness of friends and relatives outside of work, as assessed during the pre-employment period, was related to fewer symptoms. In another test, the women were categorized as belonging to three approximately equal-sized groups: the teachers (1) most exposed to work-related stressors, (2) least exposed, and (3) with intermediate levels of stressor exposures (Schonfeld, 2000). As shown in Figure 1.2, the depressive symptom levels of the three groups were indistinguishable during the pre-employment period. After school began, the most exposed teachers manifested a sharp rise in depressive symptoms. The least exposed showed a decrease in symptoms (as if a safe, well-run work environment is therapeutic). Those with intermediate exposures remained at intermediate symptom levels.

Assessing workers' characteristics before they take a job is an important idea borrowed from epidemiology. Epidemiologic researchers are concerned about selection processes leading to wrong conclusions (Berkson, 1946). In the preceding example, there is evidence that the three groups of teachers were initially equivalent on depressive symptom levels and differed only on the working conditions they were exposed to. What if hiring managers at the Board of Education (now the Department of Education) had assigned distressed teachers to the most chaotic schools and nondistressed teachers to better run schools. If the groups of teachers were not initially equivalent on levels of depressive symptoms and the investigator had not known about the lack of initial equivalence

---

9 Reverse causation in this case would mean that depressive symptoms would lead to more student-related stressors, say, by way of a depressed teacher being weak at classroom management (Schonfeld & Ruan, 1991). Later in the chapter there is a more extended discussion of reverse causation.

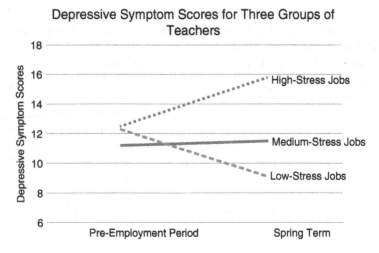

Figure 1.2 Teachers in low-, medium-, and high-stress classrooms. *Note*: The figure shows first-year women teachers' ($n = 184$) mean symptom scores on the Center for Epidemiologic Studies Depression Scale (CES-D). The sample was restricted to teachers who did not change schools between the fall and spring. The teachers were assessed before they joined the workforce (the pre-employment period) and then again during the spring term. Working conditions were assessed during the fall term. Although the pre-employment mean differences were not significant, the spring-term differences were highly significant ($p < .001$).

on the depressive-symptoms outcome variable, the investigator could have drawn conclusions based on misleading information. It is important for researchers to consider how selection processes may influence study results, including results on the impact of working conditions on depressive symptoms in teachers and other workers. Keep in mind that there are examples from the history of science that bear out the problem of selection (including research on autism[10]).

---

10 Psychiatrist Leo Kanner, who conducted pioneering research on autism, made a momentous mistake based on selection processes. He erroneously concluded that parents of autistic children are, on average, psychologically distant. But that may even have been true of the parents who brought their children to see him during the Great Depression and the beginning of World War II; it was a time when many Americans were in dire straits economically. However, mainly parents who were well-heeled enough to travel distances from their homes, disabled children in tow, could visit Kanner at Johns Hopkins University. Those observations, based on the self-selected

A lesson for longitudinal researchers who study job-related depressive symptoms is to assess and statistically control for workers' characteristics, including pre-employment depressive symptoms, when evaluating the magnitude of the link between working conditions and later symptoms. In much of the research on the impact of working conditions on depressive symptoms, we don't have, or ethically want, the ability to randomly allocate workers to more and less stressful jobs, although doing so would ensure (when using large samples) group equivalence on background characteristics. Moreover, most longitudinal research on job stress begins with workers already on the job. In that case, although not a perfect solution, it is helpful to assess key background characteristics (e.g., age, sex, initial symptom levels) along with working conditions at a study's starting point (baseline) to statistically control for variation in those characteristics when assessing the relation of baseline job conditions to later depressive symptoms. Tables 1.2 and 1.3 summarize studies that bear on the relationship of working conditions to depressive disorders or symptoms. The content of those tables is limited to studies that control for baseline disorders or symptoms when linking baseline working conditions to later disorders or symptoms.

The Demand-Control (DC) Model of Job Stress

In 1979, Robert Karasek published an important paper in the journal *Administrative Science Quarterly*. Like the article by Holmes and Rahe, Karasek's set in motion a cascade of research. This new surge in research, however, concerned the relation of working conditions to what he termed "mental strain," a label that embraced a range of problems including depressive symptoms, psychophysiologic (PP) symptoms (e.g., headaches, stomachaches, and so forth), and job dissatisfaction. He identified two

---

parents who traveled to see him, led to many psychiatrists and psychologists to conclude, wrongly, that psychological distance in parents, particularly mothers, is a key etiological factor in the development of autism (see Schonfeld & Farrell, 2010, for a fuller description). Of course, Kanner's error may look easy to identify from the vantage point of today. However, the ease with which an investigator can commit a selection-based error should not be overlooked. It took years to figure out that psychological distance in a mother does *not* cause autism. And a great deal of personal hurt to parents was done before the psychological-distance theory was put to rest.

factors that potentially affect mental strain. One he called job demands, which refers to the size of an individual's workload. The workload Karasek referred to was psychological, not physical, workload (e.g., lifting packages). Job demands or psychological workload did not only include the quantity of work but also included the extent of job complexity and the pace of work. The other factor concerned how much autonomy or control a worker has over job-related tasks.

Karasek had several intellectual forerunners. The research conducted by Friedman et al. (1958) anticipated the baleful effect of severely excessive workloads. The idea of job stressors in terms of workload also has some debt to Holmes and Rahe (1967) and Dohrenwend and Dohrenwend (1974). Also relevant to the impact of workload is that during the period from 1969 to 1977, researchers at the Institute for Social Research at the University of Michigan conducted three Quality of Employment Surveys involving representative samples of U.S. workers (Quinn & Staines, 1979). A landmark government report on the first survey (Quinn et al., 1970), largely conducted during November and December 1969, showed that one of the "foremost" job-related problems was "demands that the worker perform excessive amounts of work or work too fast" (p. 371). In addition, there were problems of monotony at work, namely, that the worker had to "do things that are very repetitious." The authors found that the intensity of work-related demands was concurrently related to reduced job satisfaction and higher levels of depressive and PP symptoms. Parallel findings emerged for workplace monotony.

Several other predecessors of Karasek were concerned with job incumbents' autonomy or control at the workplace. In 1951, the journal *Human Relations* published a paper by Eric L. Trist and Kenneth W. Bamforth. The paper concerned changes that had taken place in the British mining industry and their impact on miners.[11] The changes involved an increased division of labor and reduced autonomy for miners. Before the changes in job structure, the work of British miners had been more artisanal. The changes led to increased job dissatisfaction. Social science researchers at the University of Michigan, including Quinn and colleagues (1970),

---

11 Trist was Bamforth's mentor at the Tavistock Institute of Human Relations in London, a prestigious social science organization. Bamforth had been a miner before doing a fellowship at Tavistock. His experience represented a crack in the case-hardened British class system.

became concerned with the idea of control. Quinn et al. investigated how much "job autonomy," or, control, workers had in their positions. The study team found that autonomy was concurrently related to lower levels of depressive and PP symptoms and greater job satisfaction. The Swedish social psychologist Bertil Gardell (1971) found that the extent to which pulp and paper workers exerted control over their work tasks was directly related to better mental health. Interest in lack of control extended to psychoanalytic thinkers concerned with depression. The American psychoanalyst Edward Bibring (1953) described depression as "a state of helplessness and powerlessness of the ego" regardless of the factors that may have caused the disorder (p. 24).

Karasek's (1979) innovation was to take a combined look at workload and control (see Table 1.1). He used the term "decision latitude" in his model of job stress. The term is imbued with the idea of control. According to Karasek, decision latitude comprises two components (1) decision authority and (2) skill discretion. Decision authority refers to the extent to which the worker exerts control over meaningful job-related decisions. Skill discretion involves the diversity of job-related skills the worker can exercise. It also includes the extent to which opportunities are available to the worker to learn new skills. Mausner-Dorsch and Eaton (2000), however, advanced that view that, compared to skill discretion, decision authority is more important for mental health.

In Karasek's (1979) demand–control (DC) model of job stress, high levels of job demands "place the individual in a motivated or energized state of 'stress,'" a state that has the potential to devolve into mental strain (p. 287). However, according to the theory, decision latitude "modulates the release or transformation" of that energy into "the energy of action" (p. 287). According to the theory, there is a kind of synergy

Table 1.1 Karasek's original demand–control model.

		Job Demands	
		Low	High
Control/ Decision Latitude	Low	Passive jobs	High-strain jobs
	High	Low-strain jobs	Active jobs

between high workload and high decision latitude that benefits the worker. Karasek labeled jobs that are characterized by high demands and high control as "active jobs." In Karasek's theory, individuals holding active jobs tend to have greater opportunities for accomplishment and satisfaction as well as better mental health. An example of an active job would be that of an electrical engineer, who works hard by planning the circuitry for a new building. In an active job, the arousal precipitated by a job's demands, given the worker's control over the tasks at hand, becomes energy directed at problem-solving and goal attainment, with little arousal remaining that could become psychological strain (Karasek & Theorell, 1990).

However, for workers who face high workloads, but have little control/decision latitude, the theory holds that the worker will be at increased risk for "job strain." Jobs with high workloads and little latitude have been labeled "high-strain" jobs. An example of such a job is a worker on an assembly line. In the DC model, workers holding jobs having high workloads but with little latitude to modulate the workload's impact experience elevated levels of arousal, which gets "transformed into damaging, unused residual strain" (p. 33; Karasek & Theorell, 1990).

Apropos of high-strain jobs, it could be helpful to consider what is happening from a biological standpoint. High levels of psychosocial stressors exert effects on mental health through both the central and the autonomic nervous systems. For example, a situation in which a worker has little decision latitude when faced with high workloads or excessive job-related interpersonal conflict can challenge those systems, leading to effects such as greater catecholamine and cortisol release. Schonfeld and Chang (2017) wrote, "Stressors are interpreted by the hippocampus and amygdala and, when chronically occurring (as in high-strain jobs), can create an imbalance in allostatic (i.e., adaptive) systems such as the hypothalamic–pituitary–adrenal, or stress, axis" (p. 79). Elevated allostatic loads can have an adverse effect on mental health *and* contribute to heart disease risk by way of increased blood pressure and atherogenesis[12] (McEwen, 2004; Peters et al., 2017).

---

12 Atherogenesis refers to the forming of plaques on the innermost layer of artery walls.

To put the DC model in perspective, consider jobs characterized by high workloads combined with (1) high levels of decision latitude versus (2) low levels of decision latitude. Workers employed in high-workload, high-latitude jobs are likely to manifest fewer depressive and PP symptoms as well as greater job satisfaction. By contrast, workers employed in high-workload, low-latitude jobs are likely to manifest more depressive and PP symptoms as well as reduced job satisfaction. Thus, in the DC model, jobs that combine high workloads with high decision latitude have beneficial effects; by contrast, jobs that combine high workloads with low decision latitude have detrimental effects.

Karasek (1979) termed the type of job that combines low workload with little decision latitude a "passive job." An example of a passive job would be a watchman in a warehouse. Passive jobs, according to Karasek, lead to helplessness and, not surprisingly, passivity. The job that combines low workload with high levels of decision latitude would be termed a low-strain job. Karasek and Theorell (1990) mordantly called that type of job, if it exists, a "low-stress utopia." The authors, nonetheless, identified some occupations, based on three U.S. national surveys, as low-strain jobs. Examples they provided include lineman and natural scientist (although it would be interesting to learn how those job incumbents would respond to the low-stress/low-strain label).

One point needs to be underscored regarding Karasek's job categories. Higher socioeconomic status tends to be related to greater decision latitude and lower risk of an unfavorable effort–reward imbalance (Hoven et al., 2015; see a later section). Job categories are largely stratified along socioeconomic lines, for example, blue collar, white collar, highly educated professional, and upper management, which makes research on unraveling the impact of working conditions on depressive symptoms and disorders challenging. Are the job conditions affecting depressive symptoms in workers? Or is the socioeconomic status of job incumbents, with its attendant benefits and problems (e.g., housing conditions), affecting symptom levels? Or some combination of the two? Moreover, we need to be concerned about the influence of individuals' mental health affecting (1) the jobs they self-select, (2) hiring managers' job assignments or placement decisions, and/or (3) biases in the job incumbents' descriptions of their working conditions.

A New Development: The Demand–Control–Support (DCS) Model of Job Stress

Karasek and his colleagues (1981) extended the DC model to apply to the development of cardiovascular disease (CVD). A few years later, in connection to research on CVD, Jeffrey V. Johnson, Ellen M. Hall, and Töres Theorell (1989), when studying risk factors for CVD, introduced another dimension to the DC model, namely, social isolation, which gave rise to the "iso-strain" or demand–control–support (DCS) model. The expanded model fueled additional research.

Johnson, Hall, and Theorell's (1989) addition of social connections to the DC model has been important. Social connections already had a long history in the annals of research. The research on the health effects of social connections dates to Émile Durkheim (1951/1912), who, as mentioned earlier, linked suicide risk to upward and downward turns in the business cycle. Durkheim also found elevated suicide risk in adults who are not married. In Durkheimian thought, marriage is reflective of greater social integration. The line of research on the health-giving effects of social relationships was rediscovered and expanded with Gove (1973), Berkman and Syme (1979), and Cohen and Wills (1985). Much of the research concerned the protectiveness of family, community, and friendship ties, making it reasonable to hypothesize that socially supportive relationships with coworkers and managers are beneficial to the mental and physical health of workers. Why would supportive social relationships exert beneficial effects on mental health? At least two theoretical ideas have emerged. Supportive social relationships (1) encourage an individual, either explicitly or tacitly, to engage in adaptive health-related behaviors (e.g., encourage individuals not to smoke or give up smoking) and/or (2) have an evolutionary basis for exerting a healthful influence on the neuroendocrine axis, especially in the context of responding to stressors in the workplace and elsewhere (Schonfeld & Chang, 2017).

Moreover, research on support distinguishes between perceived and received support (Cohen & Wills, 1985; Schonfeld, 1991). Generally, the perceived availability of current support is more important to the individual's well-being. Perceived support is the pre-existing context that is available to a worker when confronted by job-related stressors. Received support tends to be confounded with prior need for support owing to previous encounters with stressful situations. In a study of new teachers, Schonfeld (2001) showed that perceived support was related to reduced levels of depressive symptoms.

The research on the DCS factors has only occasionally revealed a Karasek type of demand–control interaction. A triple interaction involving demands, control, and support is exceedingly rare. Research has tended to find that the three factors are more likely to have an additive rather than an interactive, that is, synergistic, impact on depressive symptoms. Table 1.2 bears on the impact of the DCS factors but is restricted to evidence abstracted from high-quality longitudinal studies, namely, studies that rigorously examined the impact of earlier working conditions (assessed at "Time t" or baseline) on later depressive symptoms or disorders (assessed at "Time $t + 1$") while controlling for Time t depressive symptoms or disorders. We excluded studies that failed to control for baseline depressive conditions. We also excluded studies that examined the relation of (1) change in working conditions from baseline to Time $t + 1$ to (2) change in depressive symptoms or disorders from baseline to Time $t + 1$ because such studies do not establish the temporal priority of the putative cause, working conditions, over the hypothesized effect, depressive conditions. The table demonstrates that generally workload, control, and support have an impact on depressive symptoms and disorders in the expected directions, although not perfectly consistently.

Reverse Causality

Barbara Snell Dohrenwend and Bruce Dohrenwend (1981) developed several hypothetical models of how stressful life events (SLEs) are related to changes in health symptoms. One of those models was the event proneness model, in which individuals experiencing high levels of health symptoms provoke the occurrence of SLEs. The Dohrenwends also included in the event proneness model the idea that while symptoms may provoke SLEs, those SLEs can, in turn, provoke more symptoms. The model reflects a causal relationship that is the reverse of the ordinarily expected idea that stressors provoke symptoms.

Table 1.2 High-quality longitudinal studies that bear on the relation of DCS workplace factors to depression, anxiety, and psychological distress. Parts of this table are from Schonfeld and Chang's (2017) / Springer Publishing Company. *Occupational Health Psychology: Work, Stress, and Health* by permission of the Springer Publishing Company. A key to the abbreviations is on bottom of the table.

Study team	Country	Sample	Time lag	Control variables	Major findings	Comments
Åhlin et al. (2019)	Sweden	3,947 (58% ♀)	Series of 2-yr. lags over 8 yrs.	Demographic factors + each individual as own control	Effort (demands) → ↑SCL depression Control, support ↛ depression	No evidence of reverse causality. 2-yr. lag may be too long to detect some effects.
Bromet et al. (1988)	U.S.	325 ♂'s working in power plant	1 yr.	Baseline disorder	ψWL but not DL → affective disorder by SADS and SCL-90; Unanticipated ψWL × DL interaction.	Used the GSI score from the SCL-90. Workers with less DL and greater ψWL, surprisingly, had fewer symptoms than workers with "active jobs." IVs treated as continuous variables.

Study	Country	Sample	Duration	Covariates	Findings	Notes
Bültmann et al. (2002)	Netherlands	>8,800 individuals (26% ♀)	1 yr.	Age, educ., marital status, GHQ	In ♂s, high ΨWL and emotional demands, low supervisor and coworker support, and high conflict with coworkers → ↑ GHQ but DL not significant; In ♀s, high ΨWL and emotional demands → ↑ GHQ but DL not significant	Dichotomized GHQ. Trichotomized ΨWL, demands, DL. Dichotomized support.
Burr et al. (2021)	Germany	2,212 workers; ½ ♀	5 yrs.	Age, gender, SES, baseline symptoms	Additive effects for WL and control → ↑ PHQ-9 scores; No interaction.	WL, Control, PHQ-9 dichotomized. Did not control for workers who changed jobs.
Clays et al. (2007)	Belgium	> 2,800 workers in variety of sectors (69% ♂)	6½ yrs.	Baseline CES-D	Combination of high ΨWL, low DL, and low support → incidence of ↑ CES-D scores in ♂s ΨWL, DL, and low support do not → CES-D scores in ♀s	Long follow-up likely attenuated effects. CES-D treated dichotomously. But individuals above CES-D cutoff at baseline were excluded from analyses.

(Continued)

Table 1.2 (Continued)

Study team	Country	Sample	Time lag	Control variables	Major findings	Comments
d'Errico et al. (2011)	Italy	2,046 unionized BC (80%) and WC workers (23% ♀)	5 yrs.	Age, sex	High WL → ↑ antidepressant meds prescriptions in BC workers but lowered risk in WC workers. No effect for control; No DC interaction	Excluded workers taking antidepressants at baseline. Antidepressant meds are proxy for depression. No control for job change over 5 yrs.
De Lange et al. (2004)	Netherlands	668 workers (69% ♂) The SMASH study	4 waves of data collection of 4 yrs.	Age, gender, and DV assessed in the previous wave	ΨWL affected → ↑ CES-D and EE (MBI); Control → ↑ job satisfaction; Supervisor support → ↓ EE; Job satisfaction → ↑ supervisor support; EE → ↓ supervisor support; EE → ↑ ΨWL	Predictor variables and DVs were treated as continuous factors. Used structural equation modeling that controlled for measurement error. Also found significant but weaker reverse causal effects for EE.

Author	Country	Sample	Duration	Controls/exclusions	Findings	Comments
Fandiño-Losada et al. (2013)	Sweden	4,427 workers (55% ♀) The PART Study	3 yrs.	Sociodemo., time 1 depressive symptoms	Prospective study: excluded workers with time 1 depressive dx. Poor work support → ↑ depression in ♀s ΨWL, SkD, DA ↛ depression in ♀s DA ↛ depression in ♂s ΨWL, low SkD → ↓ depression in ♂s	Dx was probable depression based on standardized questionnaire. In ♂s, finding that high ΨWL and low SkD → lower depression risk was unexpected. Among ♂s, number of cases at time 2 was low ($n = 31$; 1.5% of ♂s).
Finne et al. (2014)	Norway	3,212 workers from 48 public and private organizations (61% ♀)	2 yrs.	Age, sex, skill level Workers with high baseline symptoms excluded	Role conflict → ↑ symptoms Support from supervisor → ↓ symptoms Fair leadership → ↓ symptoms Control → ↓ symptoms only when average of baseline and follow-up used. No effect for WL	10-item symptom measure combined depressive and anxiety symptoms. Only used dichotomized (high–low) version of the symptom measure

(Continued)

Table 1.2 (Continued)

Study team	Country	Sample	Time lag	Control variables	Major findings	Comments
Juvani et al. (2018)	Finland	42,862 (80% ♀) workers from 10 towns	Until disability pension, up to 4 yrs.	Sociodemo., location, alc., smoking, hx mental and physical disorders	T1 high strain → ↑ disability pension and depression See Table 1.3	
Kawakami et al. (1992)	Japan	460 ♂, blue collar workers	4 times over 4 yrs.	Sociodemo., medical, Zung	Low control & problematic interpersonal relations → ↑ Zung High ΨWL not significant	Job's incompatibility with worker's skills → ↑ Zung. Zung scale was dichotomized.
Kivimäki et al. (2003a)	Finland	>5,600 mostly ♀ employees of 10 hospitals	2 yrs.	Sociodemo., health behaviors	High ΨWL and low DA → ↑ GHQ scores Relational justice → low GHQ scores	Trichotomized continuous IVs. Dichotomized GHQ.

Marchand et al. (2005)	Canada	National sample of > 6,000 workers (46% ♀) NHPS study	4 time points over 6 yrs.	Sociodemo.	Low DA → severe distress (6-item scale); ΨWL and support were not significant	Dichotomized continuous DV. Survival analysis to the first episode of severe distress. IVs had low reliability (e.g., ΨWL, support) and were dichotomized.
Mino et al. (1999)	Japan	310 machine workers (53% ♀)	2 yrs.	Sociodemo., excluded those with elevated baseline GHQ.	ΨWL → ↑ GHQ	Used single items to assess varieties of workload.
Niedhammer et al. (1998)	France	>11,500 workers (27% ♀) at national gas co.	1 yr.	Absenteeism owing to MH problems but not CES-D	High ΨWL, low DL, and low work-related support → ↑ CES-D	Did not control for depression at baseline. Dichotomized CES-D.
Niedhammer et al. (2015)	France	National sample 4,717 workers (≈ 50% ♂)	4 yrs.	Sociodemo., nonwork support and adversity, childhood adversity	ΨWL → GAD not MDD Emotional demands → ↑ GAD Control ↛ GAD or MDD	Prospective study. One of few studies to look at GAD dx.

(Continued)

Table 1.2 (Continued)

Study team	Country	Sample	Time lag	Control variables	Major findings	Comments
Nigatu and Wang (2018)	Alberta, Canada	2,180 (55% ♀)	4 waves, at 1-yr intervals	Sociodem., job type, history of MDD	Combo of high D/C ratio and high ERI → ↑ MDD Combo of high D/C ratio + WFC → ↑ MDD high D/C ratio alone marginally significant predictor of MDD	High D/C ratio is demand/control ratio is dichotomous. Not often used. WFC and ERI also dichotomized.
Paterniti et al. (2002)	France	>8,000 workers (75% ♂) GAZEL study	3 yrs.	Occupational grade, hostility, Type A behavior	DL, ΨWL → ↑ CES-D in ♂s ΨWL → ↑ CES-D in ♀s Work support → ↓ CES-D	IVs were measured during year 2. DV in regression was time-1–time-2 CES-D change score. Better to treat baseline CES-D as IV and time 2 CES-D as the DV.

Study	Country	Sample	Duration	Controls	Findings	Notes
Plaisier et al. (2007)	Netherlands	>2,600 workers (42% ♂) The NEMESIS study	2 yrs.	Sociodemo., physical health	Prospective study, excluded workers with disorder at baseline. ΨWL but not DL → ↑ Depressive and anxiety disorders; No effect for job security. Combined work and nonwork support → ↓ Depressive disorders	Incidence study. Used diagnostic instrument CIDI to detect disorders. ΨWL, DL, and support were continuous scales (I. Plaiser, personal communication, Nov. 11, 2014).
Rugulies et al. (2006)	Denmark	>4,100 workers (½ ♂) The DWECS study	5 yrs.	Sociodemo., health behaviors; job changing	Low supervisor support and low influence (akin to control) → ↑ depressive symptom levels in ♀s but not ♂s No effect for ΨWL.	Long follow-up likely attenuated effects (although there were statistical controls for job changes). Controlled concurrent alc., often a comorbid disorder, potentially weakening effects of IVs. DV was dichotomous. Predictors either dichotomous and/or based on single item.

(Continued)

Table 1.2 (Continued)

Study team	Country	Sample	Time lag	Control variables	Major findings	Comments
Shields (2006)	Canada NHPS study	>12,000 (≈50% ♂)	2 yrs.	Age, SES, personal stress, mastery	Strain → ↑ depression in ♂s Low coworker support → ↑ depression in ♀s	Incidence study. Depression dx by CIDI module.
Stansfeld et al. (1999)	U.K.	>7,900 civil servants (⅔ ♂) Whitehall II	5 yrs.	Sociodemo., NA, hostility, baseline GHQ or excluded those with elevated baseline GHQ	ψWL → ↑ GHQ Low DA → ↑ GHQ Low collective support → ↑ GHQ Low info from supervisor → ↑ GHQ SkD ↮ GHQ	Findings held when controlling for baseline GHQ or excluding those with high baseline GHQ.

Too et al. (2021)	Australia	1,279 (50% ♂)	4 waves over 12 yrs.	Sociodemo., verbal IQ, neuroticism, early common mental disorders	Cumulative exposure to poor job quality over first 3 waves → ↑ common mental disorder at wave 4.	Cumulative exposure = number of waves in which 2 or more of high demands, low control, and high insecurity occurred. Demands, control, and insecurity were dichotomized. Common mental disorders assessed by pattern of responses on the Goldberg scale.
Virtanen et al. (2007)	Finland	>3,300 working adults (50% ♀)	3 yrs.	Hx psycho-pathology	High ΨWL and high ΨWL × low control → affective disorder as reflected antidepressant meds prescriptions	Depression assessed by prescription for antidepressant meds. Many depressed do not take meds, and individuals with anxiety disorders sometimes take antidepressant meds.

(Continued)

Table 1.2 (Continued)

Study team	Country	Sample	Time lag	Control variables	Major findings	Comments
Wang (2004)	Canada	Same sample as Marchand et al.	4 time points over 6 yrs.	Physical health; childhood trauma; stressful life events	Low SkD, high ΨWL, low support → newly incident episode of depression	Survival model to first incidence of diagnosed depression. IVs had low reliability (e.g., ΨWL, support) and were dichotomized. Controlled contemporaneous physical health with depressive episode, likely attenuating IV-DV relation.

Note: Abbreviations: ΨWL, psychological workload or psychological demands; ♀ female; ♂ male; BC, blue collar; WC, white collar; DL, decision latitude; DA, decision authority; SkD, skill discretion; MH, mental health; NA, negative affectivity; Sociodemo., Sociodemographic variables; alc., Excessive alcohol use; CES-D, Center for Epidemiologic Studies Depression Scale; SCL-90, Symptom Checklist; MDD, major depressive disorder; GAD, generalized anxiety disorder; GSI, Global Severity Index of the SCL-90; SADS, Schedule for Affective Disorders and Schizophrenia; GHQ, General Health Questionnaire (a psychiatric symptom measure); Goldberg, Goldberg's Depression and Anxiety scales, subscales of the GHQ; Zung, Zung depression scale; hx, history; ERI, effort–reward imbalance; WFC, work–family conflict. Baseline DVs refer to the baseline versions of the dependent variables. IVs refer to the principal independent variables.

Mentioned earlier, Schonfeld (2001) in his study of New York City teachers found no evidence of reverse causality; the causal effect went exclusively from work stressors to depressive symptoms and not the other way around. In a study of Swedish workers, Åhlin et al. (2019) found no reverse causal effects for the impact of depressive symptoms on control, workload, support, and so forth, but their two-year lags may have been too long to detect such effects (details summarized in Table 1.2). In a four-year study with one year between waves of data collection, De Lange et al. (2004) in a study of Dutch workers (see Table 1.2) found no reverse effect of depression on demands, control, and support; the team, however, found emotional exhaustion, a core symptom dimension of burnout (see Chapter 2) that was assessed at the Time 1 baseline, predicted more demands and less support at Time 2, controlling for baseline demands and support.

In research on life stress, there is evidence that depressed individuals are at risk of generating new stressors (Hammen, 2020), and the research also suggests "that stress generation leads to further depression" (p. 333), thus echoing the Dohrenwends' earlier event stress proneness model. Most of the studies of workplace stress and health focus, rightfully so, on the impact of job stressors on depressive conditions and other health effects. It would still be helpful to develop a more rounded picture of the stress process by building tests of reverse causal hypotheses into analyses. The idea of reverse causal effects re-emerges in Chapter 2.

The Effort-Reward Imbalance (ERI) Model

In addition to the DCS model, several alternative models have been developed to explain the impact of work-related stressors. Among these models are the job-demands–resources, stimulus–response, conservation of resources, allostatic load, and hindrance–challenge models (Cunningham et al., 2023) as well as the person–environment fit model (Schonfeld & Chang, 2017). While this chapter is concerned with documenting the impact of adverse working conditions on depressive symptoms and disorders, none of these alternative models has generated as much high-quality longitudinal research as the DCS model. However, one other theoretical model, the effort–reward imbalance (ERI) model, runs a close second. The ERI model is therefore the only other model of job stress covered in this chapter.

In 1996, the German sociologist Johannes Siegrist published an article describing the ERI model of job stress. The ERI model rests on a long tradition in sociology and social psychology, a tradition that recognizes that the foundation of social life is group membership and exchange. Work is a socially sanctioned exchange. In exchange for a worker's efforts fulfilling the demands of a job, the worker receives benefits. What a worker applies to a job is an amalgam of effort and motivation. The motivation can be extrinsic, like pay and advancement opportunities, and/or intrinsic—enjoyment of the work itself. Leading up to the ERI model are important ideas associated with Marcel Mauss, George Homans, and Alvin Gouldner. Mauss (1954/1925), who was Émile Durkheim's nephew, showed that the giving of gifts is virtually universal. Gift-giving, in turn, creates a sense of indebtedness in the receiver, giving rise to an obligation to reciprocate. Gift-giving between groups builds alliances and social solidarity. For Homans (1958), virtually all social behavior is based on "an exchange of goods, material and non-material" (p. 597). When each person in a dyad finds the behavior of the other person reinforcing, they continue to engage with each other. When the behaviors in the dyad are not reinforcing, the dyad weakens. Gouldner (1960) advanced the view that reciprocity is a universal behavioral norm. Norms are "rules or expectations that determine and regulate appropriate behavior within a culture, group, or society" (Open Education Sociology Dictionary, 2024). Reciprocity is observed in all human societies, like, for example, the incest taboo. Gouldner wrote that the norm of reciprocity has two components: "(1) people should help those who have helped them, and (2) people should not injure those who have helped them" (p. 171). An implication of Goulder's view is that a violation of the norm of reciprocity is destabilizing.

Siegrist (1996) adapted his intellectual forebears' ideas to the work role. Accordingly, Siegrist held that disruptions to the "continuity of crucial social roles," like the work role, adversely affect the individual's self-regulatory functioning, sense of mastery, and self-esteem, giving rise to psychological distress. Layoffs, job insecurity, jobs with no opportunities for advancement, and work in which meager rewards are incommensurate with the worker's effort cause distress. Siegrist (2004) wrote that "effort at work is spent as part of a contract based on the norm of social reciprocity where rewards are provided in terms of money, esteem, and career opportunities including job security" (p. 1484). Contracts, however, are often asymmetric, to the detriment of the worker. Siegrist (1996) wisely addressed the often-posed question of why workers stay in jobs in which they face a chronic imbalance between effort and reward. He observed that many workers remain in jobs that pay low wages and offer few tangible benefits because they face high costs in quitting when there are few opportunities to obtain jobs with better conditions (e.g., pay, work–life balance).

Like the high-quality longitudinal research generated by the DC and DCS models, the ERI model has also stimulated high-quality research. Table 1.3 summarizes much of that research. As in the previous table, Table 1.3 demonstrates the adverse impact of stressful job conditions on depression and depressive symptoms in workers. Moreover, the research documented in both Tables 1.2 and 1.3 is consistent with earlier meta-analyses[13] and reviews that show the adverse effect of stressful working conditions on depressive symptoms (Bonde, 2008; Nieuwenhuijsen et al., 2010; Stansfeld & Candy, 2006; Theorell et al., 2015).

Workplace Bullying

Workplace bullying is another important stressor with adverse mental-health effects on workers. By bullying, we refer to a situation characterized by "one or more perpetrators with a power advantage over their victim systematically directing hostile behaviors toward their target over a sustained period of time" (Schonfeld & Chang, 2017, p. 164). In Nielsen and Einarsen's (2012) theoretical model, repeated exposure to workplace bullying leads to prolonged cognitive and physiological activation that results in impaired mental and physical health. In their "stress-as-offense-to-self" model, Semmer et al. (2007) advanced the view that being a target of psychological aggression at work wears down

---

13 Meta-analyses provide a way of averaging study results. We discuss meta-analyses in a footnote in Chapter 2 and again in the text of Chapter 5.

Table 1.3 High-quality longitudinal studies that bear on the relationship of the ERI model of workplace factors to depressive symptoms. Parts of this table are from Schonfeld and Chang's (2017) / Springer Publishing Company. *Occupational Health Psychology: Work, Stress, and Health* by permission of the Springer Publishing Company. A key to the abbreviations is on bottom of the table.

Study team	Country	Sample	Time lag	Control variables	Major findings	Comments
Godin et al. (2005)	Belgium	<2,000 (½ ♂) SOMSTRESS study	1 yr.	Sociodem., threat from global economy, job dissatisfaction, workplace instability	In ♂s combo of no ERI at T1 but ERI at T2 → ↑T2 depression, anxiety, somatization, and fatigue. In ♀s, combo of ERI at T1 and T2 → ↑ T2 depression, anxiety, somatization, and fatigue.	Dimensions of SCL-90 treated dichotomously. Excluded workers with above-cutoff SCL-90 scores T1 scores. Part of the effect is concurrent.
Halonen et al. (2019)	Sweden	3239 (47.5% ♀)	3 waves, waves 2 yrs. apart	Sociodemo., chronic disease, and physical WL. Excluded those with high depression scores	T1 ERI → ↑ T2 depression symptoms Part of study of depression symptoms mediating relation of ERI to neck/shoulder pain. Depression symptoms were a mediator.	Depression symptoms were continuous. ERI turned into a dichotomy.

Hoven et al. (2015)	11 Euro. countries	2798 (59% ♂)	2 yrs.	Sociodemographics, low symptom levels at baseline	T1 ERI → ↑ T2 depression symptoms ERI mediates relation of social position to depression symptoms	Not clear that all participants remained in same job over the 2 yrs. of the study.
Juvani et al. (2018)	Finland	42,862 (80% ♀) workers from 10 towns	Until disability pension, up to 4 yrs.	Sociodemo., location, alc. smoking, hx mental and physical disorders	T1 ERI → ↑ disability pension depression T1 ERI + high strain job → ↑ disability pension depression (greater effect)	ERI and high strain were dichotomized. Add organizational injustice and effect was larger.

(Continued)

Table 1.3 (Continued)

Study team	Country	Sample	Time lag	Control variables	Major findings	Comments
Kivimäki et al. (2007)	Finland	>4,800 hospital employees (Hosp. Personnel Study) + >18,000 municipal employees (10 Town Study) Mostly ♀s	2–4 yrs.	Sociodemo., employment grade.	ERI →↑ GHQ and depression dx in the 10 Town Study. ERI →↑ Depression dx in Hospital Personnel Study.	ERI comprised a single item making the findings surprising ordinarily given weaknesses of a 1-item scale. Dichotomized GHQ used in both studies. Self-reported doctor dx of depression and GHQ used in both studies. Excluded individuals with disorder or borderline disorder at baseline.
Lamy et al. (2013)	France	1,209 ♀ nurses and 908 ♀ nursing assistants	2 yrs.	Age, work unit specialty, schedule Excluded ♀s with high T1 CES-Ds	ERI →↑ depression symptoms	The T1 cutoff on the CES-D for excluding ♀s from the analyses was high, 20. Lower score like 16 would be preferable.

Study	Location	Sample	Duration	Controls	Findings	Notes
Matthews et al. (2022)	U.S.	1,599 workers (51% ♀); representative of workforce	9 yrs.	Sociodemo., alc., LTPA, job control, family problems. Excluded people with baseline depression	ERI (either as categorical or continuous variable) → ↑ risk dx of depressive episode	Family problems include excessive conflict, demands, criticism. MDE dx with CIDI. Over 9 yrs. job conditions could change. Healthy worker effect: over 9 yrs. people with unrewarding jobs could have left job or dropped out of study.
Niedhammer et al. (2015)	France	National sample 4,717 workers (≈ 50% ♂)	4 yrs.	See Table 1.2	Low reward → GAD and MDD	Prospective study. One of few studies to look at GAD.
Nigatu and Wang (2018)	Alberta, Canada	2180 (55% ♀)	4 waves, at 1-yr intervals	Sociodemo., job type, history of MDD	ERI alone → ↑ MDD Combo of high D/C ratio and hi ERI → ↑ MDD Combo of WFC and hi ERI → ↑ MDD	High D/C ratio is demand/control ratio is dichotomous. Not often used. WFC and ERI also dichotomized.

(Continued)

Table 1.3 (Continued)

Study team	Country	Sample	Time lag	Control variables	Major findings	Comments
Rugulies et al. (2013)	Denmark	Representative workforce sample 2,710 (51% ♀)	5 yrs.	Sociodemo, smoking, self-rated health, LTPA, alc.	Although ERI is most unfavorable in highest occupational grades, ERI → ↑ severe depression symptoms, with stronger impact in lower occupational grades.	Excluded individuals with high levels of depression symptoms at T1. Also controlled for continuous measure of T1 depression symptoms. Can't control for change in job conditions over time.
Stansfeld et al. (1999)	U.K.	>7,300 civil servants (⅔ ♂) Whitehall II	5 yrs.	T1 GHQ, employment grade, age	ERI → ↑ GHQ, poor social functioning, and worse general mental health	Dichotomized continuous DV. Trichotomized ERI. Excluded baseline cases of hi GHQ.

Note: Abbreviations. ERI, effort–reward imbalance; sociodemo., sociodemographic variables at baseline; ♀, female; ♂, male; LTPA, leisure time physical activity; ERI, effort–reward imbalance; GAD, generalized anxiety disorder; CES-D, Center for Epidemiologic Studies Depression Scale; hx, history; alc., excessive alcohol use; WFC, work–family conflict; D/C ratio, demand/control ratio; GHQ, General Health Questionnaire (a psychiatric symptom measure); CIDI, Composite International Diagnostic Interview; MDD, major depressive disorder; MDE, major depressive episode; T1, Time 1 and T2, Time 2. Baseline DVs refer to the baseline version of the dependent variable. IVs refer to the principal independent variables.

the victim's feelings of self-worth. Self-worth is an important personal resource, whereas reduced self-worth is a symptom of depression.

Kivimaki at al. (2003b), in a longitudinal study of more than 5,400 Finnish workers, found that job-related bullying is related to increased risk of clinical depression. Nielsen et al. (2012) in another longitudinal study, this one involving Norwegian workers ($n = 1,775$), found that having been a victim of workplace bullying is related to later increases in depressive and anxiety symptoms. In their meta-analysis, Nielsen and Einarsen (2012) found that bullying predicts later adverse mental health outcomes, including increased depressive, anxiety, and burnout symptoms. They also noted that earlier poorer mental health in workers predicts them becoming targets of bullying later. It is possible that aggressive coworkers and customers detect vulnerability in already-affected workers, which in turn arouses those potential aggressors to bully the affected workers. The issue of whether witnessing workplace bullying affects health in a substantial manner remains open to question (Nielsen et al., 2024).

Underestimates

The research summarized in Tables 1.2 and 1.3 demonstrates that workplace stressors affect depression risk, whether reflected in a diagnosable disorder or higher scores on a symptom scale. Two factors, however, suggest that the results in the two tables are underestimates of the impact of job stressors on depression. First, Altman and Royston (2006) wrote that "dichotomising a variable at the median reduces power by the same amount as would discarding a third of the data" (p. 1080). Of course, dichotomizing by pitting the highest tertile or highest quartile against everyone else also reduces a study's power to detect effects.[14] The authors recommend avoiding converting continuous variables into binary categories because of the distortion such conversions may produce. Many of the scales used in the studies in the tables,

---

14 Altman and Royston are also careful to note that sometimes when researchers hunt for an "optimal" cutoff, they risk obtaining an overestimate of the relationship between two variables, which is not the case in the studies summarized in Tables 1.2 and 1.3. Those studies tended to use arbitrary cutoffs, such as the highest quartile versus everyone else.

however, have been converted from continuous to categorical measures (dichotomized, trichotomized, etc.). It is a procrustean but popular procedure in research on depression, probably because of the ease with which results can be presented. It is often done to establish landmarks. Take, for example, a study of blood pressure; researchers are interested in identifying risk factors for hypertension. If we have two groups comprising individuals with high and low blood pressures, someone whose pressure is just below the threshold for joining the high blood pressure category is treated as equivalent to someone whose blood pressure is very good for the person's age. Consider depressive symptoms, the subject of this chapter. Researchers may regard certain cutoffs like the score of 16 on the Center for Epidemiologic Studies Depression Scale (CES-D) as an important landmark denoting high levels of distress or depression risk (Radloff, 1977). However, studying the impact of working conditions on depression by employing binary categories is problematic. A worker obtaining a depression score (1) below a cutoff (between 0 and 15 on the CES-D) or (2) at or above a cutoff (from 16 to 60) ignores all the variation scores below and above the cutoff.

In the previous paragraph, we considered endpoint variables like blood pressure and depressive symptoms. Consider now predictor variables like age. We can study the correlation of age with general physical health. What if we have a sample of adults between ages 18 and 90 and use the median to divide the sample into two groups that we call young and old? The size of the correlation between the predictor age and health is going to be smaller than if we consider age in all its variation. A similar idea applies to the predictor variables we have been discussing, predictors such as ERI and the intensity of job demands. By taking continuous measures of predictor variables and chopping them into, say, binary variables, information is lost. For example, workers in the highest quartile of job demands are pitted against everyone else. If the highest quartile is used as a marker of high workloads, the worker with a score just above that marker is considered categorically different from a worker whose score is just below that quartile marker. And the worker whose score is just a hair's breadth below the highest-quartile marker is considered a member of the same category as a worker with a relatively undemanding job. In dichotomizing (or trichotomizing) predictors (job stressors) and outcomes (depressive symptoms) the loss of information is great, thus distorting the size of the effect, usually downward.

Second, there is a selection phenomenon known as the "healthy worker effect." While the idea behind the phenomenon has long been known to epidemiologists, the term itself was coined by McMichael (1976). McMichael used the term to refer to the fact that employed individuals tend to have more favorable standardized mortality ratios (an epidemiologic measure of mortality risk) than the general population. People who have jobs are ordinarily healthy enough to work. The idea, however, does not have to be limited to mortality experience, which is why the "healthy worker effect" bears on the studies summarized in Tables 1.2 and 1.3. Individuals who are included in a worker sample are likely to be healthier than those who are not included. Furthermore, individuals included in a longitudinal study and who made it to the study's endpoint are likely to be healthier than same-age coworkers who dropped out or retired, sometimes because of the deleterious health impact of job stressors. Thus, chances are that the workers who took part in the foregoing studies were healthier than those who did not. The healthy worker effect likely reduces the size of the estimate of the impact of job stressors on depressive symptoms (e.g., Christ et al., 2007) as well as symptoms of burnout (e.g., Schaufeli, 1995).

Conclusions

Depression is a health-related problem that contributes heavily to the global burden of disease and disability (James et al., 2018). It has been recognized from the dawn of the recorded word, beginning with the *Gilgamesh* saga, the Bible, and Hippocrates. That recognition continued through the time of Shakespeare. Although it has gone by different names, thinkers as diverse as Adam Smith, Karl Marx, and Émile Durkheim have recognized it in one way or another. Depression, of course, became the subject of psychiatry, as we have represented in the work of Emil Kraepelin, Adolf Meyer, and Sigmund Freud. Investigators have come to regard depression in two different ways. One way is as a diagnosis. The other way is as a phenomenon that exists on a continuum, like temperature, with individuals who are at the high end of the continuum expected to meet criteria for a diagnosis.

The evidence presented in this chapter shows that adverse working conditions contribute to depressive symptoms and disorders. These working conditions include excessive workloads, little control over job tasks, unsupportive coworkers, imbalances disfavoring workers in terms of the efforts they put into a job and the rewards they receive from it, and bullying. Moreover, the effects described in the chapter tend to be underestimates.

Postscript

To be perfectly clear, we do *not* claim that stressful working conditions are the only contributors to depressive symptoms and disorders. We recognize that other factors contribute to depressive conditions. For example, stressful life events occurring outside the workplace can also increase the risk of clinical depression and elevated levels of depressive symptoms.

We recognize that heredity also plays a role in the development of both MDD and depressive symptoms. Sullivan et al.'s (2000) meta-analysis of twin studies shows that monozygotic in comparison to dizygotic twins[15] are more concordant for major depression, evidence that genes play a role in the disorder's emergence. Although we could not find a meta-analysis purely devoted to depressive symptoms in adults, Bergen et al.'s (2007) meta-analysis of research on adolescents and young adults indicates that there is greater similarity in depressive symptom scores between pairs of monozygotic twins compared to the similarity between pairs of dizygotic twins. Such a finding suggests that genes contribute to the emergence of depressive symptoms. While genetic influences are certain to exist, Levinson (2013) wrote "Of the three major psychiatric disorders in adults—schizophrenia, bipolar disorder, and major depressive disorder—major depression has proven to be the most challenging for modern genetic methods. This is perhaps not surprising, given that major depression is the most common and the most influenced by non-genetic factors" (p. 396). Those nongenetic factors include stressful working conditions.

---

15 Monozygotic, or identical, twins share 100% of the same genes. By contrast, dizygotic, or fraternal, twins share 50% of the same genes, like ordinary siblings.

References

Abraham, K. (1968/1911). Notes on the psychoanalytic investigation and treatment of manic-depressive insanity and allied conditions. In *Selected papers of Karl Abraham, M.D.* (pp. 127–157). D. Bryan & A. Strachey (trans.). The Hogarth Press.

Abramson, L. Y., Metalsky, G. I., & Alloy, L. B. (1989). Hopelessness depression: A theory-based subtype of depression. *Psychological Review, 96*(2), 358–372. https://doi.org/10.1037/0033-295X.96.2.358

Abramson, L. Y., Seligman, M. E., & Teasdale, J. D. (1978). Learned helplessness in humans: Critique and reformulation. *Journal of Abnormal Psychology, 87*(1), 49–74. https://doi.org/10.1037/0021-843X.87.1.49

Åhlin, J. K., LaMontagne, A. D., & Magnusson Hanson, L. L. (2019). Are there bidirectional relationships between psychosocial work characteristics and depressive symptoms? A fixed effects analysis of Swedish national panel survey data. *Occupational and Environmental Medicine, 76*(7), 455–461. https://doi.org /10.1136/oemed-2018-105450

Alloy, L. B., Abramson, L. Y., Whitehouse, W. G., Hogan, M. E., Panzarella, C., & Rose, D. T. (2006). Prospective incidence of first onsets and recurrences of depression in individuals at high and low cognitive risk for depression. *Journal of Abnormal Psychology, 115*(1), 145–156. https://doi.org/10.1037/0021-843X.115.1.145

Altman, D. G., & Royston, P. (2006). The cost of dichotomising continuous variables. *British Medical Journal, 332*(7549), 1080. http://dx.doi.org/10.1136/bmj.332.7549.1080

American Psychiatric Association. (2013). *Diagnostic and statistical manual of mental disorders,* (5th ed.). Author.

American Psychiatric Association. (2022). *Diagnostic and statistical manual of mental disorders,* 5e text rev. Author.

Beck, A. T. (2019). A 60-year evolution of cognitive theory and therapy. *Perspectives on Psychological Science, 14*(1), 16–20. https://doi.org/10.1177/1745691618804187

Beck, A. T., & Hurvich, M. S. (1959). Psychological correlates of depression: I Frequency of "masochistic" dream content in a private practice sample. *Psychosomatic Medicine, 21*, 50–55. https://doi.org/10.1097/00006842-195901000-00007

Beck, A. T., & Ward, C. H. (1961). Dreams of depressed patients: Characteristic themes in manifest content. *Archives of General Psychiatry*, *5*, 462–467. https://doi.org/10.1001/archpsyc.1961.01710170040004

Bergen, S. E., Gardner, C. O., & Kendler, K. S. (2007). Age-related changes in heritability of behavioral phenotypes over adolescence and young adulthood: A meta-analysis. *Twin Research and Human Genetics*, *10*(3), 423–433. https://doi.org/10.1375/twin.10.3.423

Berkman, L. F., & Syme, S. L. (1979). Social networks, host resistance, and mortality: A nine-year follow-up study of Alameda County residents. *American Journal of Epidemiology*, *109*(2), 186–204. https://doi.org/10.1093/oxfordjournals.aje.a112674

Berkson, J. (1946). Limitations of the application of fourfold table analysis to hospital data. *Biometrics Bulletin*, *2*(3), 47–53.

Bianchi, R., & Schonfeld, I. S. (2020). The Occupational Depression Inventory: A new tool for clinicians and epidemiologists. *Journal of Psychosomatic Research*, *138*, 110249. https://doi.org/10.1016/j.jpsychores.2020.110249

Bibring, E. (1953). The mechanism of depression. In P. Greenacre (Ed.), *Affective disorders: Psychoanalytic contributions to their study* (pp. 33–48). International Universities Press.

Bloch, A. M. (1978). Combat neurosis in inner-city schools. *American Journal of Psychiatry*, *135*, 1189–1192. https://doi.org/10.1176/ajp.135.10.1189

Bonde, J. P. E. (2008). Psychosocial factors at work and risk of depression: A systematic review of the epidemiological evidence. *Occupational and Environmental Medicine*, *65*(7), 438–445. https://dx.doi.org/10.1136/oem.2007.038430

Bromet, E. J., Dew, M. A., Parkinson, M. S., & Schulberg, H. C. (1988). Predictive effects of occupational and marital stress on the mental health of a male work force. *Journal of Organizational Behavior*, *9*, 1–13. https://doi.org/10.1002/job.4030090102

Brown, G., & Harris, T. (1978). *The social origins of depression: A study of psychiatric disorder in women*. The Free Press.

Bültmann, U., Kant, I., Kasl, S. V., Beurskens, A. J. H. M., & van den Brandt, P. A. (2002). Fatigue and psychological distress in the working population: Psychometrics, prevalence, and correlates. *Journal of Psychosomatic Research*, *52*(6), 445–452. https://doi.org/10.1016/S0022-3999(01)00228-8

Burr, H., Müller, G., Rose, U., Formazin, M., Clausen, T., Schulz, A., Berthelsen, H., Potter, G., d'Errico, A., & Pohrt, A. (2021). The demand–control model as a predictor of depressive symptoms-interaction and differential subscale effects: Prospective analyses of 2212 German employees. *International Journal of Environmental Research and Public Health*, *18*(16). https://doi.org/10.3390/ijerph18168328

Christ, S. L., Lee, D. J., Fleming, L. E., LeBlanc, W. G., Arheart, K. L., Chung-Bridges, K., Caban, A. J., & McCollister, K. E. (2007). Employment and occupation effects on depressive symptoms in older Americans: Does working past age 65 protect against depression? *The Journals of Gerontology: Series B: Psychological Sciences and Social Sciences*, *62*(6), S399–S403. https://doi.org/10.1093/geronb/62.6.S399

Clays, E., De Bacquer, D., Leynen, F., Kornitzer, M., Kittel, F., & De Backer, G. (2007). Job stress and depression symptoms in middle-aged workers—prospective results from the Belstress study. *Scandinavian Journal of Work, Environment & Health*, *33*(4), 252–259. https://doi.org/10.5271/sjweh.1140

Cobb, S., & Rose, R. M. (1973). Hypertension, peptic ulcer, and diabetes in air traffic controllers. *Journal of the American Medical Association*, *224*, 489–492. https://doi.org/10.1001/jama.1973.03220170019004

Cohen, S., & Wills, T. A. (1985). Stress, social support, and the buffering hypothesis. *Psychological Bulletin*, *98*(2), 310–357. https://doi.org/10.1037/0033-2909.98.2.310

Cruden, R. L. (1932, March 16). The great Ford myth. *The New Republic*, pp. 6–9.

Cunningham, C. J. L., Mazzola, J., & Vosika, E. C. (2023, Nov.). Stressing the theory: A systematic review and evaluation of the quality of dominant work-related stress models and frameworks. *15th International Conference on Work, Stress, and Health*.

d'Errico, A., Cardano, M., Landriscina, T., Marinacci, C., Pasian, S., Petrelli, A., & Costa, G. (2011). Workplace stress and prescription of antidepressant medications: A prospective study on a sample of Italian workers. *International Archives of Occupational and Environmental Health*, *84*(4), 413–424. https://doi.org/10.1007/s00420-010-0586-3

de Lange, A. H., Taris, T. W., Kompier, M. A. J., Houtman, I. L. D., & Bongers, P. M. (2004). The relationships between work characteristics and mental health: Examining normal, reversed and reciprocal relationships in a 4-wave study. *Work & Stress, 18*(2), 149–166. https://doi.org/10.1080/02678370412331270860

De Raedt, R., & Hooley, J. M. (2016). The role of expectancy and proactive control in stress regulation: A neurocognitive framework for regulation expectation. *Clinical Psychology Review, 45*(18), 45–55. https://doi.org/10.1016/j.cpr.2016.03.005

Dohrenwend, B. P. (1979). Stressful life events and psychopathology: Some issues of theory and method. In J. E. Barret, E. M. Rose, & G. L. Klerman (Eds.), *Stress and mental disorder* (pp. 1–15). Raven.

Dohrenwend, B. P. (2006). Inventorying stressful life events as risk factors for psychopathology: Toward resolution of the problem of intracategory variability. *Psychological Bulletin, 132*(3), 477–495. https://doi.org/10.1037/0033-2909.132.3.477

Dohrenwend, B. P., Link, B. G., Kern, R., Shrout, P. E., & Markowitz, J. (1987). Measuring life events: The problem of variability within event categories. In B. Cooper (Ed.), *The Epidemiology of Psychiatric Disorders* (pp. 103–119). Johns Hopkins Press.

Dohrenwend, B. P., Shrout, P. E., Egri, G., & Mendelsohn, F. S. (1980). Nonspecific psychological distress and other dimensions of psychopathology: Measures for use in the general population. *Archives of General Psychiatry, 37*, 1229–1236. http://dx.doi.org/10.1001/archpsyc.1980.01780240027003

Dohrenwend, B. S. (1973). Social status and stressful life events. *Journal of Personality and Social Psychology, 28*(2), 225–235. http://doi.org/10.1037/h0035718

Dohrenwend, B. S., & Dohrenwend, B. P. (1974). *Stressful Life Events: Their Nature and Effects*. John Wiley.

Dohrenwend, B. S., & Dohrenwend, B. P. (1981). Life stress and illness: Formulation of the issues. In B. S. Dohrenwend & B. P. Dohrenwend (Eds.), *Stressful life events and their contexts* (pp. 1–27). Prodist.

Durkheim, É. (1951/1912). *Suicide: A study in sociology*. In J. A. Spaulding & G. Simpson (Transl.). Free Press.

Durkheim, É. (1984/1893). *The division of labor in society*. In W. D. Halls (Trans.). Free Press.

Ellis, A. (1958). Rational psychotherapy. *Journal of General Psychology, 59*, 35–49. https://doi.org/10.1080/00221309.1958.9710170

Endicott, J., & Spitzer, R.L. (1978). A diagnostic interview: The Schedule for Affective Disorders and Schizophrenia. *Archives of General Psychiatry, 35*(5). 837–844. http://doi.org/10.1001/archpsyc.1978.01770310043002

Fandiño-Losada, A., Forsell, Y., & Lundberg, I. (2013). Demands, skill discretion, decision authority and social climate at work as determinants of major depression in a 3-year follow-up study. *International Archives of Occupational and Environmental Health*, *86*(5), 591–605. https://doi.org/10.1007/s00420-012-0791-3

Fawcett, J. A. (2013). Contributions of the NIMH collaborative depression study to *DSM–5*. In M. B. Keller, W. H. Coryell, J. Endicott, J. D. Maser, & P. J. Schettler (Eds.), *Clinical guide to depression and bipolar disorder: Findings from the Collaborative Depression Study* (pp. 203–210). American Psychiatric Publishing.

Figgis, M. (Director), Green, R. (Writer), & Burgess, M. (Writer). (2004, May 9, first broadcast). Cold cuts (Season 5, Episode 10) [TV series episode]. In D. Chase, M. Burgess, B. Grey, I.S. Landress, T. Van Patten, & T. Winter [Executive Producers], *The Sopranos*. HBO, Chase Films, and Brad Grey Television.

Finne, L. B., Christensen, J. O., & Knardahl, S. (2014). Psychological and social work factors as predictors of mental distress: A prospective study. *PLoS ONE*, *9*(7), e102514. http://dx.doi.org/10.1371/journal.pone.0102514

Freud, S. (1953–1974/1899). The interpretation of dreams (second part). *The standard edition of the complete psychological works of Sigmund Freud* (vol. 5), James Strachey (Trans. & Ed.). The Hogarth Press and The Institute of Psycho-Analysis.

Freud, S. (1953–1974/1917). Mourning and melancholia. In *The standard edition of the complete psychological works of Sigmund Freud* (vol. 14), James Strachey (Trans. & Ed.). The Hogarth Press and The Institute of Psycho-Analysis.

Friedman, M., Rosenman, R. H., & Carroll, V. (1958). Changes in the serum cholesterol and blood clotting time in men subjected to cyclic variation of occupational stress. *Circulation*, *17*, 852–861. http://doi.org/10.1161/01.CIR.17.5.852

Gardell, B. (1971). Alienation and mental health in the modern industrial environment. In L. Levi (Ed.), *Society, stress and disease* (Vol. 1, pp. 148–180). Oxford University Press.

Godin, I., Kittel, F., Coppieters, Y., & Siegrist, J. (2005). A prospective study of cumulative job stress in relation to mental health. *BMC Public Health*, *5*(67). https://doi.org/10.1186/1471-2458-5-67

Gouldner, A. W. (1960). The norm of reciprocity: A preliminary statement. *American Sociological Review*, *25*(2), 161–178. https://doi.org/10.2307/2092623

Gove, W. R. (1973). Sex, marital status, and mortality. *American Journal of Sociology*, *79*(1), 45–67. http://doi.org/10.1086/225505

Grahek, I., Shenhav, A., Musslick, S., Krebs, R. M., & Koster, E. H. W. (2019). Motivation and cognitive control in depression. *Neuroscience & Biobehavioral Reviews*, *102*, 371–381. https://doi.org/10.1016/j.neubiorev.2019.04.011

Halonen, J. I., Lallukka, T., Virtanen, M., Rod, N. H., & Magnusson Hanson, L. L. (2019). Bi-directional relation between effort–reward imbalance and risk of neck-shoulder pain: Assessment of mediation through depressive symptoms using occupational longitudinal data. *Scandinavian Journal of Work, Environment & Health*, *45*(2), 126–133. https://doi.org/10.5271/sjweh.3768

Hammen, C. (2020). Stress generation and depression. In K. L. Harkness & E. P. Hayden (Eds.), *The Oxford handbook of stress and mental health* (pp. 331–347). Oxford University Press.

Harris, T., Brown, G.W., & Bifulco, A. (1986). Loss of parent in childhood and adult psychiatric disorder: The role of lack of adequate parental care. *Psychological Medicine*, *16*(3), 641–659. https://doi.org/10.1017/S0033291700010394

Haslam, N., Holland, E., & Kuppens, P. (2012). Categories versus dimensions in personality and psychopathology: A quantitative review of taxometric research. *Psychological Medicine*, *42*, 903–920. https://doi.org/10.1017/s0033291711001966

Hawkins, N. G., Davies, R., & Holmes, T. H. (1957). Evidence of psychosocial factors in the development of pulmonary tuberculosis. *American Review of Tuberculosis*, *75*(5), 768–780. https://doi.org/10.1164/artpd.1957.75.5.768

Hempel, C. (1961). Introduction to problems of taxonomy. In J. Zubin (Eds.), *Field studies in the mental disorders* (pp. 3–22). Grune & Stratton.

Hippocrates. (1931). *Aphorisms* W.H.S. Jones (Trans.). Loeb Classical Library. Harvard University Press.

Holmes, T. H., & Rahe, R. H. (1967). The social readjustment rating scale. *Journal of Psychosomatic Research*, *11*(2), 213–218. https://doi.org/10.1016/0022-3999(67)90010-4

Homans, G. C. (1958). Social behavior as exchange. *American Journal of Sociology*, *63*, 597–606. https://doi.org/10.1086/222355

Hoven, H., Wahrendorf, M., & Siegrist, J. (2015). Occupational position, work stress and depressive symptoms: A pathway analysis of longitudinal

SHARE data. *Journal of Epidemiology and Community Health, 69*(5), 447–452. https://doi.org/10.1136/jech-2014-205206

Jackson, S. (1986). *Melancholia and depression: From Hippocratic times to modern times.* Yale University Press.

Jahoda, M., Lazarsfeld, P. F., & Zeisel, H. (1971/1933). *Marienthal: The sociography of an unemployed community.* Aldine.

James, S. L., Abate, D., Abate, K. H., Abay, S. M., Abbafati, C., Abbasi, N., Abbastabar, H., Abd-Allah, F., Abdela, J., Abdelalim, A., Abdollahpour, I., Abdulkader, R. S., Abebe, Z., Abera, S. F., Abil, O. Z., Abraha, H. N., Abu-Raddad, L. J., Abu-Rmeileh, N. M. E., Accrombessi, M. M. K., ... Murray, C. J. L. (2018). Global, regional, and national incidence, prevalence, and years lived with disability for 354 diseases and injuries for 195 countries and territories, 1990–2017: A systematic analysis for the Global Burden of Disease Study 2017. *Lancet, 392*(10159), 1789–1858. https://doi.org/10.1016/S0140-6736(18)32279-7

Johnson, J. V., Hall, E. M., & Theorell, T. (1989). Combined effects of job strain and social isolation on cardiovascular disease morbidity and mortality in a random sample of the Swedish male working population. *Scandinavian Journal of Work, Environment & Health, 15*, 271–279. https://doi.org/10.5271/sjweh.1852

Juvani, A., Oksanen, T., Virtanen, M., Salo, P., Pentti, J., Kivimäki, M., & Vahtera, J. (2018). Clustering of job strain, effort—reward imbalance, and organizational injustice and the risk of work disability: A cohort study. *Scandinavian Journal of Work, Environment & Health, 44*(5), 485–495. https://doi.org/10.5271/sjweh.3736

Karasek, R. A. (1979). Job demands, job decision latitude, and mental strain: Implications for job redesign. *Administrative Science Quarterly, 24*(2), 285–308. https://doi.org/10.2307/2392498

Karasek, R. A., Baker, D., Marxer, F., Ahlbom, A., & Theorell, T. (1981). Job decision latitude, job demands, and cardiovascular disease: A prospective study of Swedish men. *American Journal of Public Health, 71*(7), 694–705.

Karasek, R., & Theorell, T. (1990). *Healthy work: Stress, productivity, and the reconstruction of working life.* Basic Books.

Kasl, S. V. (1987). Methodologies in stress and health: Past difficulties, present dilemmas, future directions. In S. V. Kasl & C. L. Cooper (Eds.), *Stress and health: Issues in research methodologies* (pp. 162–189). Wiley.

Kasl, S. V., & Cobb, S. (1970). Blood pressure changes in men undergoing job loss: A preliminary report. *Psychosomatic Medicine, 32*(1), 19–38. https://doi.org/10.1097/00006842-197001000-00002

Kawakami, N., Haratani, T., & Araki, S. (1992). Effects of perceived job stress on depressive symptoms in blue-collar workers of an electrical factory in Japan. *Scandinavian Journal of Work, Environment & Health, 18*(3), 195–200. https://doi.org/10.5271/sjweh.1588

Kendler, K. S., & Aggen, S. H. (2023). A population-based twin study of the symptomatic diagnostic criteria for major depression that occur within versus outside of major depressive episodes. *Psychological Medicine, 53*(15), 7458–7465. https://doi.org/10.1017/S0033291723001241

Kivimäki, M., Elovainio, M., Vahtera, J., & Ferrie, J. E. (2003a). Organisational justice and health of employees: Prospective cohort study. *Occupational and Environmental Medicine, 60*(1), 27–33. https://doi.org/10.1136/oem.60.1.27

Kivimäki, M., Vahtera, J., Elovainio, M., Virtanen, M., & Siegrist, J. (2007). Effort-reward imbalance, procedural injustice and relational injustice as psychosocial predictors of health: Complementary or redundant models? *Occupational and Environmental Medicine, 64*(10), 659–665. https://doi.org/10.1136/oem.2006.031310

Kivimäki, M., Virtanen, M., Vartia, M., Elovainio, M., Vahtera, J., & Keltikangas-Järvinen, L. (2003b). Workplace bullying and the risk of cardiovascular disease and depression. *Occupational and Environmental Medicine, 60*(10), 779–783. https://doi.org/10.1136/oem.60.10.779

Kotov, R., Krueger, R. F., Watson, D., Achenbach, T. M., Althoff, R. R., Bagby, R. M., Brown, T. A., Carpenter, W. T., Caspi, A., Clark, L. A., Eaton, N. R., Forbes, M. K., Forbush, K. T., Goldberg, D., Hasin, D., Hyman, S. E., Ivanova, M. Y., Lynam, D. R., Markon, K., ::: Zimmerman, M. (2017). The hierarchical taxonomy of psychopathology (HiTOP): A dimensional alternative to traditional nosologies. *Journal of Abnormal Psychology, 126*(4), 454–477. https://doi.org/10.1037/abn0000258

Lamy, S., De Gaudemaris, R., Lepage, B., Sobaszek, A., Caroly, S., Kelly-Irving, M., & Lang, T. (2013). The organizational work factors' effect on mental health among hospital workers is mediated by perceived effort–reward imbalance: Result of a longitudinal study. *Journal of Occupational and Environmental Medicine, 55*(7), 809–816. https://doi.org/10.1097/JOM.0b013e31828acb19

Levi, L. (1972). Stress and distress in response to psychosocial stimuli: Laboratory and real life studies on sympathoadrenomedullary and related reactions. *Acta Medica Scandinavica, 528*(Suppl.), 1–166.

Levinson, D. F. (2013). Genetics of depression. In D. S. Charney, J. D. Buxbaum, P. Sklar, & E. J. Nestler (Eds.), *Neurobiology of mental illness*, (4th ed., pp. 396–410). Oxford University Press. https://doi.org/10.1093/med/9780199934959.003.0030

Linder, M., & Nygaard, I. (1998). *Void where prohibited: Rest breaks and the right to urinate on company time*. Cornell University Press.

Liu, R. T. (2016). Taxometric evidence of a dimensional latent structure for depression in an epidemiological sample of children and adolescents. *Psychological Medicine, 46*(6), 1265–1275. https://doi.org/10.1017/S0033291715002792

Liu, R. T., Kleiman, E. M., Nestor, B. A., & Cheek, S. M. (2015). The hopelessness theory of depression: A quarter century in review. *Clinical Psychology: Science and Practice, 22*(4), 345–365. https://doi.org/10.1111/cpsp.12125

Marchand, A., Demers, A., & Durand, P. (2005). Do occupation and work conditions really matter? A longitudinal analysis of psychological distress experiences among Canadian workers. *Sociology of Health & Illness, 27*(5), 602–627. https://doi.org/10.1111/j.1467-9566.2005.00458.x

Marx, K. (1967/1844). Economic and philosophical manuscripts. In L. D. Easton & K. H. Guddat (Eds. & Trans.), *Writings of the young Marx on philosophy and society* (pp. 283–337). Anchor Books.

Matthews, T. A., Porter, N., Siegrist, J., & Li, J. (2022). Unrewarding work and major depressive episode: Cross-sectional and prospective evidence from the U.S. MIDUS study. *Journal of Psychiatric Research, 156*, 722–728. https://doi.org/10.1016/j.jpsychires.2022.11.009

Mausner-Dorsch, H., & Eaton, W. W. (2000). Psychosocial work environment and depression: Epidemiologic assessment of the demand-control model. *American Journal of Public Health, 90*, 1765–1770. https://doi.org/10.2105/AJPH.90.11.1765

Mauss, M. (1954/1925). *The gift: Forms and functions of exchange in archaic societies*. In I. Cunnison (Trans.). Coehn & West.

McEwen, B. S. (2004). Protection and damage from acute and chronic stress: Allostasis and allostatic overload and relevance to the pathophysiology of psychiatric disorders. *Annals of the New York Academy of Sciences, 1032*, 1–7. https://doi.org/10.1196/annals.1314.001

McMichael, A. J. (1976). Standardized mortality ratios and the "healthy worker effect": Scratching beneath the surface. *Journal of Occupational Medicine, 18*(3), 165–168.

Mino, Y., Shigemi, J., Tsuda, T., Yasuda, N., & Bebbington, P. (1999). Perceived job stress and mental health in precision machine workers of Japan: A 2 year cohort study. *Occupational and Environmental Medicine, 56*(1), 41–45. https://doi.org/10.1136/oem.56.1.41

Monroe, S. M., Bromet, E. J., Connell, M. M., & Steiner, S. C. (1986). Social support, life events, and depressive symptoms: A 1-year prospective study. *Journal of Consulting and Clinical Psychology, 54*(4), 424–431. https://doi.org/10.1037/0022-006X.54.4.424

Moscarello, J. M., & Hartley, C. A. (2017). Agency and the calibration of motivated behavior. *Trends in Cognitive Sciences, 21*(10), 725–735. https://doi.org/10.1016/j.tics.2017.06.008

Niedhammer, I., Goldberg, M., Leclerc, A., Bugel, I., & David, S. (1998). Psychosocial factors at work and subsequent depressive symptoms in the Gazel cohort. *Scandinavian Journal of Work, Environment & Health, 24*(3), 197–205. https://doi.org/10.5271/sjweh.299

Niedhammer, I., Malard, L., & Chastang, J.-F. (2015). Occupational factors and subsequent major depressive and generalized anxiety disorders in the prospective French national SIP study. *BMC Public Health, 15*, 200. https://doi.org/10.1186/s12889-015-1559-y

Nieuwenhuijsen, K., Bruinvels, D., & Frings-Dresen, M. (2010). Psychosocial work environment and stress-related disorders, a systematic review. *Occupational Medicine, 60*(4), 277–286. https://doi.org/10.1093/occmed/kqq081

Nielsen, M. B., & Einarsen, S. (2012). Outcomes of exposure to workplace bullying: A meta-analytic review. *Work & Stress, 26*(4), 309–332. https://doi.org/10.1080/02678373.2012.734709

Nielsen, M. B., Einarsen, S. V., Parveen, S., & Rosander, M. (2024). Witnessing workplace bullying—A systematic review and meta-analysis of individual health and well-being outcomes. *Aggression and Violent Behavior, 75*, 101908. https://doi.org/10.1016/j.avb.2023.101908

Nielsen, M. B., Hetland, J., Matthiesen, S. B., & Einarsen, S. (2012). Longitudinal relationships between workplace bullying and psychological distress. *Scandinavian Journal of Work, Environment, & Health, 38*(1), 38–46. https://doi.org/10.5271/sjweh.3178

Nigatu, Y. T., & Wang, J. (2018). The combined effects of job demand and control, effort–reward imbalance and work-family conflicts on the risk of major depressive episode: A 4-year longitudinal study. *Occupational and Environmental Medicine, 75*(1), 6–11. https://doi.org/10.1136/oemed-2016-104114

Open Education Sociology Dictionary. (2024, February). https://sociologydictionary.org/norm/#definition_of_norm

Oswin, M. (1978). *Children living in long-stay hospitals*. Heinemann.

Overmier, J. B., & Seligman, M. E. (1967). Effects of inescapable shock upon subsequent escape and avoidance responding. *Journal of Comparative and Physiological Psychology, 63*(1), 28–33. https://doi.org/10.1037/h0024166

Parkes, K. R. (1982). Occupational stress among student nurses: A natural experiment. *Journal of Applied Psychology, 67*, 784–796. https://doi.org/10.1037/0021-9010.67.6.784

Paterniti, S., Niedhammer, I., Lang, T., & Consoli, S. M. (2002). Psychosocial factors at work, personality traits and depressive symptoms. Longitudinal results from the GAZEL Study. *British Journal of Psychiatry 181*, 111–117. https://doi.org/10.1192/bjp.181.2.111

Peters, A., McEwen, B. S., & Friston, K. (2017). Uncertainty and stress: Why it causes diseases and how it is mastered by the brain. *Progress in Neurobiology, 156*, 164–188. https://doi.org/10.1016/j.pneurobio.2017.05.004

Peterson, C., Maier, S. F., & Seligman, M. E. P. (1993). *Learned helplessness: A theory for the age of personal control*. Oxford University Press.

Pickles, A., & Angold, A. (2003). Natural categories or fundamental dimensions: On carving nature at the joints and the rearticulation of psychopathology. *Development and Psychopathology, 15*(3), 529–551. https://doi.org/10.1017/S0954579403000282

Plaisier, I., de Bruijn, J. G. M., de Graaf, R., ten Have, M., Beekman, A. T. F., & Penninx, B. W. J. H. (2007). The contribution of working conditions and social support to the onset of depressive and anxiety disorders among male and female employees. *Social Science & Medicine, 64*(2), 401–410. https://doi.org/10.1016/j.socscimed.2006.09.008

Popper, K. R. (1963). *Conjectures and refutations: The growth of scientific knowledge*. Harper Torchbooks.

Quinn, R. P., Seashore, S. W., Kahn, R. L., Mangone, T., Campbell, D., Staines, G. L., McCullough, M., Oliker, N., & Shulman, M. (1970). *Survey of working conditions. Final report on univariate and bivariate tables*.

Survey Research Center, The University of Michigan. U.S. Dept. of Labor Employment Standard Administration.

Quinn, R. P., & Staines, G. L. (1979). *The 1977 quality of employment survey: Descriptive statistics with comparison data from the 1960–70 and the 1972–73 surveys*. Institute for Social Research, University of Michigan.

Radloff, L. S. (1977). The CES-D Scale: A self-report depression scale for research in the general population. *Applied Psychological Measurement, 1*(3), 385–401. https://doi.org/10.1177/014662167700100306

Rahe, R. H., Meyer, M., Smith, M., Kjaer, G., & Holmes, T. H. (1964). Social stress and illness onset. *Journal of Psychosomatic Research, 8*, 35–44. https://doi.org/10.1016/0022-3999(64)90020-0

Ramazzini, B. (1700/1750). *Health preserved, in two treatises. I. On the diseases of artificers, which by their particular callings they are most liable to. With the method of avoiding them, and their cure. II. On those distempers, which arise from particular climates, situations and methods of life. With Directions for the choice of a healthy air, soil and water* (2nd ed.). R. James (Trans.). Eighteenth Century Collections Online, The British Library.

Riskind, J. H., Beck, A. T., Berchick, R. J., Brown, G., & Steer, R. A. (1987). Reliability of *DSM–III* diagnoses for major depression and generalized anxiety disorder using the Structured Clinical Interview for *DSM–III*. Archives of General Psychiatry, *44*(9), 817–820. https://doi:/10.1001/archpsyc.1987.01800210065010

Rugulies, R., Aust, B., Madsen, I. E. H., Burr, H., Siegrist, J., & Bültmann, U. (2013). Adverse psychosocial working conditions and risk of severe depressive symptoms. Do effects differ by occupational grade? *European Journal of Public Health, 23*(3), 415–420. https://doi:/10.1093/eurpub/cks071

Rugulies, R., Bültmann, U., Aust, B., & Burr, H. (2006). Psychosocial work environment and incidence of severe depressive symptoms: Prospective findings from a 5-year follow-up of the Danish work environment cohort study. *American Journal of Epidemiology, 163*(10), 877–887. https://doi.org/10.1093/aje/kwj119

Sadowsky, J. (2021). *The empire of depression: A new history*. Polity Press.

Schaufeli, W. B. (1995). A cautionary note about the cross-national and clinical validity of cut-off points for the Maslach Burnout Inventory. *Psychological Reports., 76*, 1083–1090.

Schonfeld, I. S. (1991). Dimensions of functional social support and psychological symptoms. *Psychological Medicine, 21*(4), 1051–1060. https://doi.org/10.1017/s003329170003004x

Schonfeld, I. S. (1992). Assessing stress in teachers: Depressive symptoms scales and neutral self-reports of the work environment. In J. C. Quick, L. R. Murphy, and J. J. Hurrell, Jr. (Eds.), *Work and well-being: Assessments and instruments for occupational mental health* (pp. 270–285). American Psychological Association. https://doi.org/10.1037/10116-018

Schonfeld, I. S. (1996). Relation of negative affectivity to self-reports of job stressors and psychological outcomes. *Journal of Occupational Health Psychology, 1*(4), 397–412. https://doi.org/10.1037/1076-8998.1.4.397

Schonfeld, I. S. (2000). An updated look at depressive symptoms and job satisfaction in first-year women teachers. *Journal of Occupational and Organizational Psychology, 73*(3), 363–371. https://doi.org/10.1348/096317900167074

Schonfeld, I. S. (2001). Stress in 1st-year women teachers: The context of social support and coping. *Genetic, Social, and General Psychology Monographs, 127*(2), 133–168.

Schonfeld, I. S. (2006). School violence. In E. K. Kelloway, J. Barling, & J. J. Hurrell, Jr. (Eds.), *Handbook of workplace violence* (pp. 169–229). Sage Publications. https://doi.org/10.4135/9781412976947.n9

Schonfeld, I. S., & Bianchi, R. (2022). Distress in the workplace: Characterizing the relationship of burnout measures to the Occupational Depression Inventory. *International Journal of Stress Management, 29*(3), 253–259. https://doi.org/10.1037/str0000261

Schonfeld, I. S., & Chang, C.-H. (2017). *Occupational health psychology: Work, stress, and health.* Springer Publishing Company. https://doi.org/10.1891/9780826199683

Schonfeld, I. S., & Farrell, E. (2010). Qualitative methods can enrich quantitative research on occupational stress: An example from one occupational group. In D. C. Ganster & P. L. Perrewé (Eds.), *Research in occupational stress and wellbeing series. Vol. 8. New developments in theoretical and conceptual approaches to job stress* (pp. 137–197). Emerald. https://doi.org/10.1108/S1479-3555(2010)0000008007

Schonfeld, I. S., & Ruan, D. (1991). Occupational stress and preemployment measures: The case of teachers. *Journal of Social Behavior and Personality, 6*(7), 95–114.

Schonfeld, I. S., Verkuilen, J., & Bianchi, R. (2019). An exploratory structural equation modeling bi-factor analytic approach to uncovering what burnout, depression, and anxiety scales measure. *Psychological Assessment, 31*(8), 1073–1079. http://dx.doi.org/10.1037/pas0000721

Seligman, M. E. P. (1975). *Helplessness: On depression, development, and death*. W. H. Freeman.

Seligman, M. E., & Maier, S. F. (1967). Failure to escape traumatic shock. *Journal of Experimental Psychology, 74*(1), 1–9. https://doi.org/10.1037/h0024514

Selye, H. (1956). *The stress of life*. McGraw-Hill.

Semmer, N. K., Jacobshagen, N., Meier, L. L., & Elfering, A. (2007). Occupational stress research: The "stress-as-offense-to-self" perspective. In J. Houmont & S. McIntyre (Eds.), *Occupational health psychology: European perspectives on research, education and practice* (pp. 43–60). ISMAI Publishers.

Shields, M. (2006). Stress and depression in the employed population. *Health Reports, 17*(4), 11–29.

Siegrist, J. (1996). Adverse health effects of high-effort/low-reward conditions. *Journal of Occupational Health Psychology, 1*, 27–41. http://dx.doi.org/10.1037/1076-8998.1.1.27

Siegrist, J., Starke, D., Chandola, T., Godin, I., Marmot, M., Niedhammer, I., & Peter, R. (2004). The measurement of effort-reward imbalance at work: European comparisons. *Social Science & Medicine, 58*, 1483–1499. http://dx.doi.org/10.1016/S0277-9536(03)00351-4

Smith, A. (1976/1776). *An inquiry into the nature and causes of the wealth of nations*. University of Chicago Press.

Speiser, E. A. (Trans.) (1955). *The epic of Gilgamesh*. In J. E. Pritchard (Ed.), *Ancient Near Eastern texts relating to the Old Testament with supplement*. Princeton University Press.

Stansfeld, S., & Candy, B. (2006). Psychosocial work environment and mental health—a meta-analytic review. *Scandinavian Journal of Work, Environment & Health, 32*(special issue 6), 443–462. http://dx.doi.org/10.5271/sjweh.1050

Stansfeld, S. A., Fuhrer, R., Shipley, M. J., & Marmot, M. G. (1999). Work characteristics predict psychiatric disorder: Prospective results from the Whitehall II Study. *Occupational and Environmental Medicine, 56*(5), 302–307. https://doi.org/10.1136/oem.56.5.302

Sullivan, P. F., Neale, M. C., & Kendler, K. S. (2000). Genetic epidemiology of major depression: Review and meta-analysis. *American Journal of Psychiatry, 157*(10), 1552–1562. https://doi.org/10.1176/appi.ajp.157.10.1552

The Jewish Publication Society. (1917). *The holy scriptures: According to the Masoretic Text: A new translation.* Author.

Theorell, T., Hammarström, A., Aronsson, G., Bendz, L. T., Grape, T., Hogstedt, C., Marteinsdottir, I., Skoog, I., & Hall, C. (2015). A systematic review including meta-analysis of work environment and depressive symptoms. *BMC Public Health, 15*(1), 1–14. https://doi.org/10.1186/s12889-015-1954-4

Too, L. S., Leach, L., & Butterworth, P. (2021). Cumulative impact of high job demands, low job control and high job insecurity on midlife depression and anxiety: A prospective cohort study of Australian employees. *Occupational and Environmental Medicine, 78*, 400–408. https://doi.org/10.1136/oemed-2020-106840

Tyndale House (1996). *Holy bible: New living translation.* Publisher.

Virtanen, M., Honkonen, T., Kivimäki, M., Ahola, K., Vahtera, J., Aromaa, A., & Lönnqvist, J. (2007). Work stress, mental health and antidepressant medication findings from the Health 2000 Study. *Journal of Affective Disorders, 98*, 189–197. https://doi.org/10.1186/1471-2458-12-236

Wallace, M. (2003). *The American axis: Henry Ford, Charles Lindbergh, and the rise of the Third Reich.* St. Martin's Press.

Wang, J. L. (2004). Perceived work stress and major depressive episodes in a population of employed Canadians over 18 years old. *Journal of Nervous and Mental Disease, 192*(2), 160–163.

World Health Organization. (1990). *Composite International Diagnostic Interview, Version 1.0.* Author.

World Health Organization. (2024). *Clinical descriptions and diagnostic requirements for ICD-11 Mental, behavioural and neurodevelopmental disorders.* Author.

2

Burnout

Two figures established the foundation of the burnout concept as it is known today. One is Herbert J. Freudenberger and the other, Christina Maslach. Working independently, both made the idea of burnout widely known. Before they entered the picture, there had been some prior mentions of burnout. For example, in 1961 the British writer Graham Greene published the novel *A Burnt-Out Case* about a famous architect who, repelled by the fame he acquired, goes off to the Congo to work at a leper colony. In a 1969 paper, H. B. Bradley, an associate superintendent of research for the California Department of Corrections, described an innovative, multifaceted approach to treating young adult offenders. In a single sentence, Bradley expressed the view that the new approach would offset staff burnout. Robert Sommer (1973), in an autobiographical paper entitled "The Burnt-Out Chairman," depicted the work life of a university department chairperson; his signs of burnout included his feelings of frustration in accomplishing little more than completing administrative "housekeeping chores" and symptoms such as gastrointestinal pains when a medical examination found nothing wrong. In 1974, Sigmund G. Ginsburg dedicated a brief paper to "the problem of the burned out executive" Ginsberg described burnout in terms of tensions flowing from the grind of corporate life, irritability, excess alcohol consumption, erratic decision-making (shifting between making decisions too quickly and too slowly), and casting blame for problems on others. There have probably been other mentions of burnout in books, magazines, and other media prior to

Breaking Point: Job Stress, Occupational Depression, and the Myth of Burnout, First Edition. Irvin Sam Schonfeld and Renzo Bianchi.
© 2025 John Wiley & Sons, Inc. Published 2025 by John Wiley & Sons, Inc.

the influential work of Freudenberger and Maslach. However, their efforts prompted many people to think further about work-related burnout.

Herbert J. Freudenberger

Clinical psychologist Herbert J. Freudenberger briefly mentioned burnout in a 1973 paper but described it more fully later. The concept of burnout entered the social science lexicon in 1974, when Freudenberger published a historic paper in the *Journal of Social Issues*. That paper, entitled "Staff Burn-Out," described psychological, physical, and behavioral stress-related symptoms of what many regard as burnout.

The journalist Douglas Martin (1999) wrote that Freudenberger "was no stranger to stress." Born in 1926 to a Jewish family from Frankfurt, he was pursued by gangs of Hitler youth after school (Gold Medal, 1999). In November 1938, at age 12, he saw his synagogue burn down. It was at that age that he escaped from Germany, using a fake passport, to make his way to rooming houses in a series of European cities before arriving in New York City. Once in the city, he stayed with a distant relative who mistreated him. At age 14, he lived in the streets before a cousin took him in. Resilient, he quickly learned English and later attended Brooklyn College (Canter & Freudenberger, 2001). While working at night in factories, he earned a doctorate at NYU in clinical psychology and completed training in psychoanalysis (Gold Medal, 1999). After he completed a full day of work in his private practice, he devoted himself, without pay, to establishing free clinics to help substance abusers, some of whom were Vietnam veterans.

Freudenberger (1973), writing in *Psychotherapy: Theory, Research and Practice*,[1] published what is probably the first paper that explicitly, although briefly, described burnout in a psychology/social science journal. The context of the description involved psychologists working in a free clinic in the late 1960s and early 1970s. He also admitted to having experienced the problem himself. He described burnout this way:

---

[1] The journal's name subsequently changed to *Psychotherapy*.

"You feel a total sense of commitment. The whole atmosphere builds up to it, until you finally find yourself, as I did, in a state of exhaustion and your doctor tells you that you must leave or your health will be in jeopardy." (p. 56)

Freudenberger's influential 1974 paper, "Staff Burn-Out," was based on his observations of the volunteers working at those free clinics *and* his own work in the clinics. The concept of burnout had the flavor of *bricolage* (Friberg, 2009). He could not have provided case studies, a common feature of articles about clinical phenomena, because doing so would have identified specific volunteers. Instead, he painted a broad picture of burnout. He enumerated its physical signs, which included fatigue, exhaustion, headaches, gastrointestinal problems, insomnia, and shortness of breath. Freudenberger also described burnout's behavioral signs. These included feeling overburdened when asked to complete a small task, expressing dissatisfaction with what is asked for by angrily yelling, paranoia regarding coworkers' attitudes toward other staff members, and excessive use of tranquilizers and marijuana. In describing its psychological features, Freudenberger wrote that many burned-out individuals looked as if they were depressed.

According to Freudenberger, some individuals are prone to burnout. These include staff members who, upon realizing that the individuals they were serving had tremendous needs, gave excessive and unrealistic amounts of themselves to their patients. A staff member may feel guilt for not giving enough, which feeds even more giving. Freudenberger also observed another source of burnout. He noted that, eventually, the excitement of starting a clinic wears off once funding has been established and a stable administration is in place, in which case routinization takes hold, leading some staff members to become bored. For those staff members, the monotony of the job breeds burnout.

Freudenberger (1975) described two sets of pressures that affect the individual staff member. One type is internal. The professional often feels intense self-induced pressure to succeed at addressing the desperate needs of the community members the professional is trying to serve. The other type is the pressure that comes from administrators who want the professional to give more. Then Freudenberger used the idea of those pressures to distinguish commitment and overcommitment. According to Freudenberger, the overcommitted are more likely to experience burnout.

Freudenberger did not conduct large-scale studies of burnout. He did not look for a basis for burnout in contemporary psychology or psychiatry. His observations were based on a relatively small number of people. Beginning in the 1980s, larger-scale quantitative research on burnout began to take root. Such research has the potential to yield valuable, generalizable knowledge about an entity such as burnout.

Christina Maslach

The other leading figure in establishing the foundations of the concept of burnout is Christina Maslach. After earning an undergraduate degree from Radcliffe/Harvard, she earned a PhD at Stanford. Maslach went on to become a professor of psychology at the University of California, Berkeley. Famously, she persuaded Philip Zimbardo, her former dissertation advisor and later husband, to end his notorious Stanford Prison Experiment (Zahneis, 2018).[2] Her interceding in the study is dramatized in a feature film (Alvarez, 2015).

To our knowledge, Maslach published her first article about burnout in 1976 in *Human Behavior: The Newsmagazine of the Social Sciences*. Whereas Freudenberger's 1974 paper was based on observations of his coworkers and himself, Maslach's (1976) magazine article was based on observations of 200 helping professionals, such as social workers, prison staff, psychiatric nurses, and psychiatrists, who worked intensely with patients, prisoners, clients, and others. Maslach collected data from the professionals using methods not clearly described in the article. The reliability and validity of these initial observations remain unknown to this day. Although research on burnout was just beginning, the "syndrome" is presented as if it were an established entity.

Her magazine article, echoing Freudenberger's work, reported that burned-out workers typically feel emotionally exhausted. The article began with a vignette about a burned-out poverty lawyer who became very angry with a poor client. Then going on to describe the burnout phenomenon in some detail, Maslach mentioned that the intensity of burnout differs by occupation and burnout rates are lower in professionals

---

2 While the Stanford Prison Experiment has often been criticized on ethical grounds, it has also proved problematic from a scientific standpoint (Le Texier, 2019).

who "actively express, analyze, and share their personal feelings." The reference to burnout rates is surprising because, to calculate burnout rates, it is necessary to know how to diagnose someone who is suffering from burnout and identify someone who isn't. There were no diagnostic criteria for burnout in 1976. Maslach also reported that burnout can lead to alcohol abuse, mental health problems, insomnia, ulcers, migraine headaches, and suicide, but neither evidence nor sources were presented.

This inaugural article focused largely on how burned-out helping professionals coped with job stress. According to Maslach, coping tended to take several forms of distancing from clients, children, and patients. The varieties of distancing included depersonalization, callousness, neglect of duty, giving oneself time-outs, seeking administrative jobs to get away from clients and children, and expressing disparaging views about the people the professionals were supposed to help.

The article also touched on personal accomplishment. For example, some professionals thought their feelings reflected a "personal failing" or they lacked the "interpersonal skills" necessary to succeed at the job. The sense of personal failing is evident in a poverty lawyer who said, "I was trained in law, but not in how to work with the people who would be my clients. And it was that difficulty in dealing with people and their personal problems, hour after hour, that became the problem for me, not the legal matters per se" (p. 22). Maslach noted that many health and social service workers acknowledged that their interpersonal skills were deficient.

Maslach, together with Ayala Pines, published a second article, in 1977, in the professional journal *Child Youth Care Forum*. The article concerned burnout in 83 staff members at various daycare centers. The staff members completed questionnaires that comprised both open-ended questions and psychometric scales that were cursorily described. While they summarized the results in the paper, descriptions of their statistical findings were only available upon request. Clinical case reports were also absent. In the absence of statistical findings, Maslach and Pines reported that workers at centers with higher ratios of children to staff members or who worked longer hours tended to experience more stress and dissatisfaction with their jobs. The researchers also reported that some childcare workers coped with job stressors by taking short breaks or diverting themselves to less stressful tasks such as paperwork.

Pines and Maslach (1978) described a study of burnout in 76 staff members working in mental health facilities. In the context of an interview designed for the study, the staff members responded to open-ended questions and completed psychometric scales. The authors found that higher workloads and more interaction with the most severely affected patients (e.g., those with schizophrenia) were related to greater job dissatisfaction. Although the authors mentioned that the correlations they calculated among variables of interest were statistically significant ($p < .05$), they published no correlation coefficients. In fact, they published no quantitative findings. They also wrote that "the incidence of burnout is often very high in health and social service professions" (pp. 233–234) without explaining how they assessed incidence.[3]

In 1978, Maslach published a piece in the *Journal of Social Issues*, the same journal in which Freudenberger had published his clinical observations in 1974. She identified several client factors that she suggested made work emotionally demanding. These factors included patients so severely affected that there is little chance of professional help ameliorating their conditions, bureaucratic rules that are stumbling blocks to better interactions with clients, and the abundant negative feedback a professional receives when something goes wrong in comparison to the relatively little positive feedback a professional gets when things go right. One lacuna in this fourth paper in her series is the absence of statistical findings on burnout based on the "several hundred helping professionals of various types" who contributed to the research.

Correlation Coefficients and Reliability Coefficients

Because research on burnout is quantitative in nature, we wrote this brief section to help readers who are nonspecialists better understand the material that follows. A reader who has research experience may want to skip the section.

---

3 Incidence is a term that reflects the number of individuals who represent *new* cases of a disorder divided by the total number of people in the population from which the affected individuals come, per unit of time. The unit of time could be one month, one year, or whatever unit a research team deems appropriate.

The foundations of what we know about burnout largely involve the Pearson correlation coefficient, which is symbolized by an italicized, lowercase letter r. This statistic helps us understand findings related to the validity of burnout (sub)scales. The correlation coefficient reflects the extent to which two factors are linearly related. It ranges from 0, in which there is utterly no relation between the two factors, to 1.00 (or −1.00), in which a score on one factor perfectly predicts a score on the other factor. According to a rule of thumb suggested by Jacob Cohen (1977), small correlations center around .10; medium correlations, .30; and large correlations, .50.[4] In research in psychology and psychiatry, it is relatively rare, but not unheard of, to find correlations that exceed .50.

Virtually every score on a psychological test or scale is purported to reflect an entity, called a construct, which cannot be directly observed. For example, a score on a depressive symptom scale is thought to index something inside the individual's head, namely, the intensity of the distress the individual is experiencing. However, a score on a psychological scale reflects *more* than the construct the scale is purported to measure. A certain amount of random noise or "measurement error," which is ordinarily indexed by a scale's reliability coefficient,[5] contributes to test and scale scores. A reliability coefficient can vary from 0 to 1.00. A reliability coefficient estimated to be 0 indicates that scale scores are 100% random noise. A coefficient of 1.00 suggests that there is no measurement error and that scale scores perfectly index the underlying construct. Generally, researchers are happy when reliability coefficients are greater than .80 (in which scale scores reflect 80% of the variability of the underlying construct) and even happier when they are greater than .90 (in which scale scores reflect 90% of the variability of the underlying construct).

Despite the theoretical maximum reliability of 1.00, no psychological symptom scale or any other type of psychological scale measures a

---

4 We alert readers allied to disciplines other than psychology, our not placing a zero before the decimal point is consistent with the style mainly used in our discipline, psychology, when reporting correlation coefficients. In other disciplines, for example, psychiatry, a zero is placed before the decimal point.
5 The two most popular reliability coefficients are called alpha and, no surprise, omega. The alpha coefficient has been more commonly used, although the omega coefficient is more sophisticated statistically.

construct without error. By error, we generally mean any random fluctuations that go into the measurement of a psychological construct any time a psychological scale is administered to individuals. To be clear, the concept of error in this context is *not* reflective of avoidable mistakes. The term "error" in psychometric theory was "inherited from an earlier era in psychology when interest centered on finding general laws of behavior" (Anastasi & Urbina, 1997, p. 84). Apart from flaws in scale items (e.g., confused wording), in the context in which we are using the term, "error" refers to the inevitable variability intrinsic to the measurement process.

Measurement error in two burnout subscales (or in any two psychological scales) reduces the magnitude of the correlation between the two scales. Correlation coefficients, however, can be corrected for measurement error. A method is available that allows us to estimate what a correlation between two factors could be if the factors had been measured without error (Cohen et al., 2003). That estimate is called a disattenuated or corrected correlation coefficient (which we symbolize like this: $r_{x'y'}$). Research papers typically report correlation coefficients and, only occasionally, disattenuated correlation coefficients. If authors didn't publish disattenuated correlation coefficients, readers can sometimes calculate these corrected coefficients by making use of the published correlation coefficients and the scales' reliability coefficients that authors almost always include in their writing.

A downside of researchers using the disattenuated correlation coefficient involves correlating scales in which one or both scales have low reliability coefficients. The result is that the corrected correlation coefficient is likely to be inflated in such a way as to yield a misleadingly high estimate of the true relationship being studied. A remedy for this problem is for researchers to employ scales that demonstrate high reliability.

The Foundations of Burnout

Freudenberger and Maslach's introduction of the idea of burnout to a wide audience was helpful in an important way. Although past research had addressed the impact of difficult working conditions on workers, the efforts of Freudenberger and Maslach helped to sensitize other researchers and the public to problems facing professionals such as clinicians, social workers, and teachers. Many helping professionals are excessively exposed to interactional stressors (e.g., a teacher being confronted by an aggressive student). For example, research has found that interactional stressors take a considerable toll on teachers' well-being (Schonfeld & Feinman, 2012).

At the time Freudenberger and Maslach were publishing their first papers on job-related burnout, other investigators (e.g., Brown et al., 1973; Dohrenwend, 1973) were making progress in understanding how life's stressors can give rise to psychological symptoms. Earlier research, mentioned in Chapter 1, advanced our understanding of the impact of job stressors on physical health (e.g., Friedman et al., 1958). Neither Freudenberger nor Maslach in their first publications cited any of that era's burgeoning research and theorizing on the physical or psychological impact of stressors (e.g., Selye, 1956), let alone examine the relation of earlier research and theorizing to their own observations regarding what they called burnout. Through 1981, most of their citations were references to their own work, including evanescent conference proceedings. Thus, the papers published did not include a systematic review of the literature on stress and health. That literature was essentially ignored.

In 1981, Maslach and Susan Jackson published an influential paper in the *Journal of Occupational Behaviour*. The paper was entitled "The Measurement of Burnout." It told the story of the development of the Maslach Burnout Inventory (MBI), an instrument "designed to measure the hypothesized aspects of the burnout syndrome" (p. 100). Maslach and Jackson tried out 47 potential questionnaire items on a sample of more than 600 individuals who worked in health and service occupations (e.g., police, teachers, psychiatrists, social workers). The 47 items derived from a review of previously collected questionnaire and interview data as well as content found in established scales (although not borrowed verbatim). The team subjected the responses to a factor analysis. One goal of a factor analysis is to identify underlying dimensions (potential constructs) that might explain the correlations among all or most of the items. Inspection of the results led the investigators to reduce the number of items to 25. Then Maslach and Jackson tried out these 25 items on a second group of more than 400 helping professionals.

They ultimately arrived at three underlying factors or constructs that partly explained the correlations among 22 items. They labeled the factors Emotional Exhaustion (EE), Depersonalization (DP), and (reduced) Personal Accomplishment (PA). The items that "loaded" on (i.e., correlated with) each specific factor became the items that made up the EE, DP, and PA subscales of the MBI. EE refers to the extent to which work has depleted a worker's emotional ("I feel emotionally drained from my work") and physical ("I feel fatigued when I get up in the morning") resources, limiting how much that worker can continue to devote to the job. DP refers to the extent to which a worker has developed negative and cynical attitudes, indifference, even callousness, regarding coworkers, clients, patients, and students ("I feel I treat some recipients as if they were impersonal 'objects'"). Regarding the domain of reduced PA, this subscale assesses the extent to which workers have come to negatively evaluate their own work-related competence or achievement ("I deal very effectively with the problems of my recipients"). This three-component conceptualization of burnout eventually crystallized into burnout's definition.

In view of Maslach et al.'s (2001) approach to burnout, consider that the EE subscale assesses symptoms of fatigue and loss of energy a worker ascribes to work. The fatigue and loss of energy experienced by the worker are to be conceived of both psychologically and physically. The DP subscale assesses the extent to which a worker disengages or detaches from relationships with coworkers, clients, patients, students, and others—the putative sources of stress. Their demands appear "more manageable when they are considered impersonal objects of one's work" (Maslach et al., p. 403). According to Maslach et al., depersonalizing is supposed to "protect" the worker from the emotional arousal those others can provoke. DP, thus, amounts to a form of coping with the stress- and exhaustion-producing personalities in the workplace. EE (and DP) are then likely to erode or interfere with a worker's sense of accomplishment. In the view of Maslach et al., a reduced sense of accomplishment is a result of EE (and DP). EE can thus be regarded as the nucleus of burnout.

Maslach and Jackson (1981) were concerned with the construct validity of the subscales of the MBI. As part of *construct validity*, researchers must demonstrate *convergent and discriminant validity*

(Campbell & Fiske, 1959).[6] Although we look at discriminant validity a little later, suffice it to say at this juncture that evidence of convergent validity requires that a scale purported to assess a construct (e.g., the EE subscale of the MBI) and alternate measures of the same construct be substantially correlated.

As shown in Table 2.1, Maslach and Jackson provided some evidence of convergent validity using a subgroup of 40 mental health workers. The table indicates that workers' EE scores correlated reasonably well with how a coworker rated the worker for being emotionally or physically drained. The workers' DP scores were less well correlated with the coworkers' ratings; however, the DP scores were more highly correlated with coworkers' ratings of feeling emotionally and physically drained, a kind of cross-over correlation. The results for PA were not significant and not reported.

Table 2.1 also shows the results from another component of Maslach and Jackson's (1981) convergent validity research. These findings pertain to 142 male police officers. The correlation of their EE scores with their wives' ratings of the husbands' upset and anger was moderate. The police officers' PA scores correlated less strongly with the wives' ratings of the husband for returning home from work in "a cheerful or happy mood" or the husbands' regarding police work as "a source of pride and prestige for the family." There was no reporting on DP in the police-officer sample. The findings bearing on the police-officer sample are problematic, given how imperfectly the alternative measures assessed the constructs in question. At the time of the study, most other measures of burnout (e.g., the Copenhagen Burnout Inventory, the Shirom-Melamed Burnout Measure) had not yet been developed. Because Pines et al.'s (1981) burnout measure was being developed independently of and at about the same time as the MBI, it was likely unavailable to Maslach and Jackson for the purpose of establishing the MBI's convergent validity.

---

6 There is more to establishing construct validity than demonstrating convergent and discriminant validity, but we don't want to make this chapter too technical. Suffice it say that there are other facets of construct validity. For example, it is important for psychometric researchers to demonstrate the measurement invariance of a scale, i.e., that scale items have approximately the same meaning in different demographic groups, such as males and females.

Table 2.1 Correlational findings regarding the convergent validity of the subscales of the Maslach Burnout Inventory (MBI) as excerpted from the Results section of the paper.

Variables	Alternative measure	Sample	r
EE and Emotionally Drained rating	Coworker's rating	40 mental health workers	.41
EE and Physically Drained rating	Coworker's rating	40 mental health workers	.42
DP and Emotionally Drained rating	Coworker's rating	40 mental health workers	.57
DP and Physically Drained rating	Coworker's rating	40 mental health workers	.50
DP and alternative rating	Coworker's rating	40 mental health workers	.33
PA and alternative rating	Coworker's rating	40 mental health workers	ns
EE and upset-angry	Wife's rating	140 male police officers	.34
DP	No reporting		
PA and return home happy or cheerful mood	Wife's rating	140 male police officers	.20
PA and pride-prestige for family	Wife's rating	140 male police officers	.25

Note: EE = Emotional Exhaustion subscale of the MBI; DP = Depersonalization subscale of the MBI; PA = Personal Accomplishment subscale of the MBI. Adapted from Maslach and Jackson (1981).

Three years after the publication of the MBI, another burnout instrument appeared, the Meier Burnout Assessment, which comprised 23 true–false items (e.g., "Many of the activities I once found enjoyable at work are no longer much fun"; "I have a lot of self-doubt about work").[7] Scott T. Meier (1984), using a sample of professors, showed evidence of the instrument's convergent validity. The MBI's total score, a sum of EE, DP, and reduced PA, was highly correlated with Meier's own burnout scale, $r = .61$, and the professors' self-ratings of burnout, $r = .65$.

---

7 We thank Scott T. Meier for providing us with the original instrument.

There are, however, troubling aspects to Maslach and Jackson's (1981) introduction of the MBI to the world. First, the definition of burnout reflected in the MBI was largely pre-established, that is, established prior to the MBI's 1981 publication date. With job stress, particularly interactional stressors involving clients, as the putative cause of burnout, Maslach's (1976) early original magazine article already described the "fatigue," "emotional overload," "psychological distancing and withdrawal," "cynical or negative attitudes," and "sense of personal failing" deemed to characterize burnout (see Bianchi & Schonfeld, 2023). Schaufeli and Enzmann (1998, p. 188) noted: "the MBI has been developed inductively by factor-analysing a rather arbitrary set of items. What would have happened if other items had been included? Most likely, other dimensions would have appeared!" The symptom items in the factor analyses largely reflected preconceptions found in Maslach's (1976) magazine article and in Pines and Maslach's (1978) paper. Pines and Maslach (1978) wrote, without presenting supporting data: "Burnout can be defined as a syndrome of physical and emotional exhaustion, involving the development of negative self-concept, negative job attitudes, and loss of concern and feeling for clients" (p. 233). Clearly, burnout's definition was preset.

Second, Maslach and Schaufeli (1993) acknowledged that her research on burnout did not emerge out of existing theory. We stress that there is nothing wrong per se with such an approach; it is often used in qualitative research (Schonfeld & Mazzola, 2013). However, when the early research on burnout was taking place, the burnout pioneers seemed to ignore earlier relevant contemporaneous research on stress, research conducted by Barbara and Bruce Dohrenwend and George Brown and Tirril Harris, to name a few. The burnout pioneers also ignored the research of social scientists at the University of Michigan's Institute for Social Research, who investigated the impact of job-related stressors (e.g., Caplan et al., 1975; Kahn et al., 1964).

Third, Maslach and Jackson (1981) wrote that burnout is a syndrome that comprises emotional exhaustion, depersonalization/cynicism, and reduced levels of personal accomplishment. They published the correlations among the three component burnout symptom

Table 2.2 Correlations obtained from the Results section adapted from Maslach and Jackson (1981) paper on the creation of the Maslach Burnout Inventory (MBI). The correlations involving symptom frequencies are below the diagonal and the correlations involving symptom intensity are above the diagonal.

	EE	DP	PA
EE		.50	−.05
DP	.44		−.22
PA	−.17	−.28	

Note: EE = Emotional Exhaustion subscale of the MBI; DP = Depersonalization subscale of the MBI; PA = Personal Accomplishment subscale of the MBI.

subscales—they assessed the symptoms in two ways, in terms of frequency and intensity. Table 2.2, which was constructed from what the authors published in their Results section, shows the correlations. The correlations were quite low, probably too low to reflect a syndrome. By definition, a syndrome refers to a "grouping of signs and symptoms, based on their frequent co-occurrence" (American Psychiatric Association, 2013).

Finally, the paper addressed the discriminant validity of the burnout subscales in a questionable manner. In this context, discriminant validity refers to evidence that the burnout construct is distinguishable from other psychological constructs. Maslach and Jackson (1981), using a small sample ($n = 91$), showed that the components of burnout had low correlations with job satisfaction; EE's correlation job satisfaction was −.23, surprisingly stronger than EE's correlation with PA (−.17 or −.05, depending upon whether examining frequency or intensity), again underlining the question of syndromal unity. However, a more relevant test of discriminant validity would have been to examine burnout's relation to psychological symptom scales that were in existence at the time the MBI was introduced, such as the Depression scale of the MMPI (Hathaway & McKinley, 1940); Radloff's (1977) Center for Epidemiologic Studies Depression Scale, Goldberg's (1972) General Health Questionnaire (a measure of psychological distress), or Langner's (1962) 22-item psychiatric symptom scale.

More on Discriminant Validity

Research on the discriminant validity of the MBI soon emerged after the publication of Maslach and Jackson's 1981 paper on the MBI. Meier (1984) found that a score based on the total MBI was about as highly correlated with the MMPI Depression scale ($r = .57$) as it was with Meier's own burnout scale ($r = .61$).

Early foundational studies by Leiter and Durup (1994) and Bakker et al. (2000) gave a misleading impression that burnout and depression are distinct constructs. In a study of Canadian healthcare workers, Leiter and Durup found what appeared to be evidence for the discriminant validity of the MBI vis-à-vis depressive symptoms as measured by the Beck Depression Inventory (BDI). Leiter and Durup's study was problematic because they chopped up the BDI into smaller, less reliable subscales, which would reduce the magnitude of burnout–depression correlations. However, even then EE was about as closely related to an abbreviated BDI subscale ($r = .46$) as it was to DP ($r = .47$). Leiter and Durup also employed a procedure called confirmatory factor analysis (CFA). The researchers used a CFA to estimate the correlation between the burnout and depression constructs (along with BDI items, they added items from a second measure of depressive symptoms to reflect the depression construct) with measurement error controlled (something like a disattenuated correlation, which we described earlier). They found that the burnout–depression correlation, with measurement error controlled, was quite high ($r_{xy'} = .72$). We found the authors' interpretation that the CFA provides evidence of discriminant validity problematic for two other reasons. First, the CFA had a poor model fit; in other words, it did not adequately represent the relations among the different constructs.[8] Second, Leiter and Durup did not use almost half the depressive symptom items available to them, yet the burnout–depression correlation was quite high.

In a study of Dutch teachers, Bakker et al. (2000), using the Center for Epidemiological Studies Depression scale (CES-D) and the MBI, concluded that they provided "strong evidence for the discriminant

---

8 The adjusted goodness of fit index (AGFI) was .810. An AGFI greater than .90 would have inspired greater confidence in the model they proposed.

validity of burnout and depression" (p. 261). The conclusion is problematic for at least two reasons. First, the EE core of burnout was more highly correlated with each of two truncated depressive symptom scales Bakker et al. created by breaking up the entire CES-D into shorter, hence less reliable subscales ($r = .68$ and $.56$) than with Depersonalization ($r = .47$) and Personal Accomplishment ($r = -.47$). Second, the time frame for the scale items ascertaining symptom frequency in the MBI was the past year and the time frame for symptom frequency in the CES-D was one week, a format difference that likely reduced the magnitude of the EE–depression correlation, yet the correlational evidence showed that the EE–depression relationship was stronger than the relationships among the MBI subscales. Leiter and Durup (1994) also used burnout and depression measures with incommensurate time frames.

Antecedents of Burnout

In the history of the concept of burnout, there had been some early questions regarding the factors that contribute to its development. Maslach (1993) wrote that at the heart of burnout are emotionally demanding, interactional stressors. By contrast, in their review of the literature available at the time, Schaufeli and Enzmann (1998) found that workload-related stressors are more closely related to burnout than caregiving stressors. They referred to factors such as high workloads, time pressure, and role conflict. For example, they observed that hospital doctors found time pressures more stressful than working with seriously ill patients. The authors concluded that "on empirical grounds, the assertion that burnout is particularly related to emotionally charged interactions with clients has to be refuted" (p. 84).

Schaufeli and Enzmann (1998) also reviewed personality-related antecedents of burnout. The leading personality factor among the antecedents was neuroticism. Neuroticism is considered a broad and fundamental dimension of personality that reflects a propensity to experience negative, distressing emotions (e.g., dysphoric mood, anxiety, anger/hostility, and helplessness) and to exhibit the associated cognitions and behaviors (e.g., low self-esteem, inhibition of action). The authors also noted that one other personality factor, hardiness, is (inversely) related to burnout.

Hardiness is a composite of three elements: control, commitment, and challenge (Kobasa, 1979). Control involves the extent to which individuals believe that they can exert some control or influence over life's events. Commitment refers to the depth or extent to which individuals involve themselves in life's activities. Challenge refers to individuals' ability to feel positive excitement when confronting change. The antecedents, whether personality variables or work-related factors, were more closely related to EE than to the other two components of burnout.

While Schaufeli and Enzmann's (1998) review of the literature identified some "antecedents" of burnout, most of the findings should be regarded with caution because the studies they reviewed were largely cross-sectional (Enzmann, 2005). From a cross-sectional study, we only know that factor A and factor B covary with each other actuarially. We don't know if they correlate with each other because A caused B or B caused A. One of the criteria to be met for a causal inference to be made is that the cause temporally precedes the effect. We also don't know if A and B correlate with each other because some unmeasured third factor(s) caused both.

Longitudinal studies are helpful because we can ensure temporal precedence of the putative cause over the putative effect. Schaufeli and Enzmann (1998) reported on eight longitudinal studies that evaluated the effect of baseline work stressors on later burnout controlling for baseline burnout. They found scant evidence that work stressors cause burnout. The directionality of the hypothesized stressors-to-burnout effect was largely wrong. In other words, Schaufeli and Enzmann found evidence of reverse causality, that EE at Time 1 was related to higher work demands at Time 2, statistically controlling for Time-1 demands.

We will return to the theme of job stressors causing burnout versus burnout causing job stressors toward the end of the chapter, when we examine meta-analyses conducted many years later, at a time when more longitudinal research on burnout had been conducted.

The Multiplication of Burnout Scales

Beginning with the publication of the MBI in 1981, investigators developed other measures of burnout. That same year, Pines and her colleagues published a 21-item burnout scale (the instrument had a different name when first published; we will report on the scale in Chapter 3). As previously mentioned, Meier (1984) also created a burnout scale. Maslach and her colleagues developed several variants of the original MBI (Maslach et al., 1996; 2016). For example, they created the MBI-General Survey (MBI-GS), which was designed to be used with a larger cross-section of occupations (sample item: "I feel used up at the end of the workday."). The subscales of the MBI-GS were a little different from the original MBI, which applied only to the helping professions. The MBI-GS subscales are named Exhaustion, Cynicism, and Professional Efficacy.

One or another variant of the MBI has been employed in almost 90% of the published articles bearing on burnout (Schaufeli et al., 2009; Schonfeld et al., 2019). Schonfeld et al. found that many of the remaining articles have been about equally divided among three non-MBI burnout scales: the Oldenburg Burnout Inventory (Demerouti et al., 2001), the Shirom-Melamed Burnout Measure (Shirom & Melamed, 2006), and the Copenhagen Burnout Inventory (Kristensen et al., 2005a).

The Oldenburg Burnout Inventory (OLBI), in comparison to the MBI, has more of a foundation in theory (sample item: "There are days when I feel tired before I arrive at work."). In developing the OLBI, Demerouti et al. (2001) reformulated the concept of burnout based on their theoretical model of job stress, the job demands–resources (JD–R) model. Schonfeld and Chang (2017) described the model in some detail, explaining that it was an expansion of the demand–control–support model, which was described in Chapter 1. In the JD–R model, job demands refer to the physical (e.g., heavy lifting), social (e.g., argumentative customers), and/or mental demands (e.g., the complexity of work problems) that are part of a job. Job resources can be external or internal (Demerouti et al., 2001). Examples of external resources include an organizational structure that fosters worker control over tasks, supportive coworkers, and helpful equipment (e.g., devices that minimize lifting). Examples of internal resources include a worker's cognitive ability and accumulated past learning. The idea behind the OLBI is that higher levels of job demands lead to exhaustion and lower levels of job resources contribute to disengagement from the job. Thus, the OLBI comprises two subscales, Exhaustion and Disengagement. An innovation of the OLBI is that negatively and positively worded items are interlaced through the subscales, which likely inclines users to pay closer attention to the items, reducing careless responding.[9] Although the OLBI was deemed to assess burnout, in practice it assesses two constructs, exhaustion and disengagement. Like the MBI, the OLBI does not produce a total burnout score.

The Shirom-Melamed Burnout Measure (SMBM; sample item: "I feel tired.") is also connected to a theoretical model, namely Hobfoll's (1989) conservation of resources (COR) theory. COR theory also contributed to the JD–R model. The idea behind COR theory is that people are motivated to obtain, retain, and protect their resources (Hobfoll & Shirom, 2001). Examples of resources include relationships with others, job connections, and personal characteristics such as self-esteem. Schonfeld and Chang (2017) underlined the asymmetrical nature of COR theory, namely, that "All things being equal, resource loss is psychologically more injurious to a person than resource gain is beneficial to the individual" (p. 90). In developing the SMBM, Shirom and Melamed (2006) concentrated on one set of resources—energetic resources. Energy plays a central role in the individual's well-being. Energy depletion is a drag on other resources. Shirom and Melamed also aimed to differentiate the SMBM from the MBI by removing references to coping with exhaustion (e.g., depersonalization, distancing from others) and the consequences of exhaustion (e.g., reduced accomplishment).

Dissatisfied with the MBI, Kristensen et al. (2005a) developed the Copenhagen Burnout Inventory (CBI; sample item: "Do you feel worn out at the end of the working day?"). They expressed dissatisfaction with the idea that "Burnout is what the MBI measures, and the MBI measures what burnout is" (p. 193). One of the factors that motivated Kristensen et al. to create the CBI was that with the MBI "we have one concept but three independent measures" (p. 194). In other words, they criticized the fact that the MBI reflects three separate entities and not a unified construct—burnout. Kristensen et al., like Shirom and Melamed, recognized that reduced accomplishment is more a consequence of exhaustion than a part of burnout, and depersonalization/distancing is a coping strategy. Finally, Kristensen et al. criticized the MBI because it is not in the public domain. That is to say, unlike the case of the CBI, SMBM, and OLBI, which are freely available, a researcher must pay to use the MBI.

---

9 In the scoring, the positively worded items get reverse scored.

Our focus here is on the work-related version[10] of the CBI, which can be completed by most job incumbents. Although Kristensen et al. (2005a) underlined Maslach and colleagues having been atheoretical in developing the MBI, the development of the CBI was similarly atheoretical. Building on the "historical development of the burnout concept," Kristensen et al. defined work-related burnout as *"The degree of physical and psychological fatigue and exhaustion that is perceived by the person as related to his/her work"* (authors' italics, p. 196). The scale underlines the causal attributions people make regarding the connection of each symptom to work. Items from the CBI have been incorporated into the Copenhagen Psychosocial Questionnaire, a comprehensive instrument created for assessing occupational risk factors and the connection between work and health (Burr et al., 2019; COPSOQ International Network, 2024; Kristensen, 2010; Kristensen et al., 2005b). The questionnaire, including CBI items, has been translated into more than 25 languages.

To conclude this section, we underline that the World Health Organization (WHO, 2022) endorsed a definition of burnout that reflects the content of the MBI. Importantly, the WHO does not treat burnout as a medical or psychiatric diagnosis, but as an "occupational phenomenon." Alternative instruments involve alternative definitions of burnout. This state of affairs illustrates the persistent difficulties encountered by burnout researchers in agreeing on the basic nature of their entity of interest.

Problems with Burnout Symptom Items That Are Synonymous

The use of expressions that are synonymous or near-synonymous with each other in essays and literature can sometimes enliven writing or add clarity to complex texts. However, in scale construction, synonymy can be problematic. Although seemingly harmless, an over-reliance on

---

10 Another version of the CBI is dedicated for use by professionals who have clients, but the word "client" can be replaced with "student" or "patient" if desired. A third version assesses "personal burnout," which applies to anyone, an employed person, an unemployed individual, a retired person, and so on.

near-synonymous items in scale construction can create the illusion that a scale is better than it actually is.

There is considerable synonymy in the MBI EE subscale. For example, the MBI EE subscale includes such near-synonymous items as "Working with people all day is really a strain for me" and "Working with people directly puts too much stress on me." This pattern of near-synonymy also holds true for other burnout scales. For example, the Cognitive Weariness subscale of the SMBM contains these items: "I have difficulty concentrating," "I feel I am not thinking clearly," and "I feel I am not focused on my thinking." Scale reliability, an important psychometric quality that contributes to a scale's validity, depends on correlations among the items the scale comprises, that is, item-to-item agreement. Having many items within a scale that are synonymous or near-synonymous increases item-item correlations, giving a "patina of reliability" (Bianchi, Verkuilen, et al., 2023), thus making the scale appear more attractive to practitioners than it ought to be.

To put the foregoing problem of synonymy in perspective, consider this contrast. The PHQ-9, a depressive symptom scale with robust psychometric properties (Bianchi, Verkuilen, et al., 2022), differs from the previously mentioned burnout scales regarding the use of synonymy. The PHQ-9 assesses symptoms of depression. The scale's items (e.g., depressed mood, appetite disturbance, suicidal ideation) show no explicit synonymy (Bianchi, Verkuilen, et al., 2023), and yet the scale has excellent reliability. The PHQ-9 has excellent reliability because the scale's items assess different facets of one underlying construct without depending on superficial similarities in item wording. What binds those symptom items together is that they reflect the underlying construct, namely, depression. Much of what binds together the items on burnout scales is the overreliance on synonymy.

Burnout as a Diagnosis

Many researchers have treated burnout as a diagnostic entity. Maslach (1976) did it implicitly when she wrote that "burnout rates" are lower in some professionals than in others. Maslach and Leiter (1997) did it too when claiming that "[b]urnout is reaching epidemic proportions among North American workers today" (p. 1). To refer to burnout rates or epidemics means that there is a way to identify cases of burnout. Of course, Maslach has not been alone in mentioning burnout rates, that is, estimates of burnout prevalence. To assess the prevalence of burnout, we need to have a way of diagnosing it, which would enable us to indicate that one person meets criteria for a diagnosis and another does not. To date, however, no clear and consensual diagnostic criteria for burnout exist.

Diagnostic confusion has prevailed in burnout research from its inception. In the absence of sound diagnostic criteria for burnout, investigators have generally relied on identification criteria that are clinically and theoretically arbitrary as well as heterogeneous. In a systematic review of 182 studies pertaining to physician burnout, Rotenstein et al. (2018) found "at least 142 unique definitions for meeting overall burnout or burnout subscale criteria" (p. 1144). In the absence of sound diagnostic criteria, it is advisable to suspend judgment on whether burnout is a widespread condition.

Longitudinal Research on Adverse Working Conditions and Burnout

Three etiologically oriented meta-analyses (Aronsson et al., 2017; Guthier et al., 2020; Lesener et al., 2019) shed some light on the relationship of adverse working conditions to burnout. To estimate those averages, the meta-analysts assembled pertinent primary studies. Aronsson et al. employed a fixed-effects model, Lesener et al. a random-effects model, and Guthier et al. both.[11] Each meta-analysis

---

11 To arrive at an average correlation or regression coefficient (we will call both an effect size), each coefficient extracted from a primary study is, to some extent, weighted by the size of that study's sample. In studies that generate regression coefficients, such as the studies by Aronsson et al. and Guthier et al., the meta-analytic procedures are used to average these coefficients, which reflect, for example, the relation of job stressors at the Time 1 to burnout symptoms at Time 2. The weighting of the contributions of the primary studies differs depending upon whether a researcher conducts a random- or fixed-effects meta-analysis (Borenstein et al., 2021). Briefly, in a fixed-effects model, the researcher assumes that one "true" effect size underlies the variation in the effect sizes found in the primary studies. Any variation in the effect sizes reflects sampling error. A summary effect in the fixed-effects model, which is an estimate of the true effect size, is the weighted average of the effects extracted from the primary studies.

evaluated the average strength of the longitudinal relation of baseline (Time-1) working conditions to later (Time-2) burnout. Because of their importance, we will chronologically examine each of the foregoing meta-analyses in some depth.

Aronsson et al. (2017)

Guided by the demand–control–support model (described in Chapter 1), Aronsson et al. identified 25 longitudinal studies and experiments as well as studies that they deemed the "equivalent" of longitudinal analyses (e.g., case-control studies[12]). Using those studies, the investigators conducted a meta-analysis for the purpose of assessing the link between adverse working conditions and later burnout. Burnout was defined as present or absent, as if it were a diagnosis. Instead of producing correlations, the studies produced adjusted odds ratios. An odds ratio (*OR*) is a measure of the association between exposure to a risk factor and a medical or psychological outcome.[13] In this study, the *OR* was adjusted

---

In the random-effects model, the analyst assumes that, rather than there being one true effect, true effects themselves vary from sample to sample. Sampling error (as in the fixed-effects model) also contributes to variation among effect sizes. Borenstein et al. wrote, "If it were possible to perform an infinite number of studies (based on the inclusion criteria for our analysis), the true effect sizes for these studies would be distributed about some mean" (p. 59). In the random-effects model, the analyst assumes that the effect sizes found in the primary studies are a random sample of all the possible effect sizes. In the fixed-effects model, averaging of effect sizes is weighted by a study's sample size with the goal of estimating a summary effect that is the "true" effect size. By contrast, a goal of a random-effects meta-analysis is *not* to estimate one true effect size, but to estimate the mean of all the true effect sizes. In the random-effects model, effect sizes from larger samples carry larger weights but not as large as in fixed-effects models; smaller samples have larger weights than found in fixed-effects models. Also see Chapter 5.

12 A case-control study includes at least two groups, individuals who have a "disorder" (in this case burnout) and comparison individuals without the disorder. The research team compares the groups on past exposure to risk factors such as high workloads (either represented as a categorical variable such as high- or low-workload or workload as assessed on a continuum). Usually, sociodemographic and other factors (e.g., other exposures) are statistically controlled or controlled by matching.

13 For example, if the prevalence of burnout is 2% in the individuals unexposed to a key risk factor (RF) such as low control and the OR = 1.5, then the prevalence of burnout in those exposed to the RF would be about 50% greater or approximately 3.0%. If the *OR* = 2, then the prevalence in the exposed individuals would be about

statistically for the influence of potential confounding factors (e.g., sociodemographic factors).

Based on nine studies, Aronsson et al. found that low job control at baseline was significantly related to later EE ($OR = 1.63$). Based on 13 studies, high levels of psychological job demands were related to later EE ($OR = 2.53$). Four studies linked psychological demands to depersonalization/cynicism ($OR = 2.37$). The study team also found that low workplace support (nine studies; $OR = 1.81$) predicted EE. Reduced PA was too rarely studied to be reported on. Some of the studies used continuous measures of burnout scales and converted the results to bear on present–absent outcomes (see Chapter 1 for problems concerning dichotomizing). Other problems with the meta-analysis included the diagnostic heterogeneity of burnout (Rotenstein et al., 2018) and the mixing together of longitudinal and less well-controlled case-control studies.

Lesener et al. (2019)

As the framework for their meta-analysis, Lesener et al. employed the job demands–resources (JD–R) model, which we discussed earlier in this chapter. With the JD–R model as their framework, physical, social, and organizational job demands, for example, time pressures, role conflicts, and workload, are thought to have psychological and physiological costs. Resources, such as autonomy, support, and equipment, refer to aspects of the job that function to help workers successfully complete job-related tasks and attain related goals. Lesener et al. calculated the average correlations among the variables based on the aggregated studies. They built structural regression models[14] based on the average correlations among Time-1 and Time-2 burnout,

---

100% greater or approximately 4%. We use the words "about" and "approximately" because *ORs* are affected by several factors, including the prevalence of the outcome in the sample being studied, that make the estimates approximations.

14 In nontechnical terms, multiple regression/correlation provides a means to study how several factors predict an outcome variable. It informs us how the factors perform in concert in predicting the outcome and how each factor does separately in predicting the outcome, statistically controlling (adjusting) for the influence of the other factors.

demands, and resources. Based on a structural regression, the authors found that Time-1 job demands predicted increased Time-2 burnout symptoms and Time-1 job resources decreased Time-2 symptoms, statistically controlling for Time-1 burnout.

The study team published a table showing the correlations they calculated based on averages obtained from between 28 and 44 samples. We concentrate on the part of the table that pertains to burnout's exhaustion core, rather than job engagement, which Lesener et al. also reported on. We reconstructed their table to include job demands, job resources, and burnout assessed at the Time-1 baseline and at Time 2 (see Table 2.3). While the matrix shows that resources and demands assessed at baseline predicted Time-2 burnout, the table also shows that burnout at Time 1 was related to demands and resources at Time 2.

We used the correlation matrix in Table 2.3 to further explore how Time-1 factors related to Time-2 burnout. We note, however, that Lesener et al.'s structural regression model was based on correlations that were aggregated over many studies. Consequently, their regression results do not necessarily apply to, and are probably stronger than, the relationships at the level of the individual participants in the primary

Table 2.3 Correlation matrix excerpted from the meta-analysis conducted.

	Resources T1	Demands T1	Burnout T1	Burnout T2	Resources T2
Demands T1	−.20				
Burnout T1	−.32	.41			
Burnout T2	−.28	.36	.65		
Resources T2	.61	−.15	−.25	−.37	
Demands T2	−.15	.62	.34	.48	−.20

Note: T1 refers to Time 1 or the baseline measurement period; T2 refers to the Time 2 follow-up period. According to Lesener et al., all correlations were significant, $p < .001$. Adapted from Lesener et al. (2019).

studies.[15] With that caveat in mind, we proceeded to conduct a multiple regression analysis. But note that not every correlation was calculated in every sample employed in Lesener et al.'s meta-analysis. For example, 43 samples provided correlations between job demands and job resources at Time 1 but 37 provided correlations between demands at Time 1 and burnout at Time 2. We ran our own regression analysis because we were primarily interested in an alternate test of how demands and resources at Time 1 related to burnout at Time 2.

With the correlations in Table 2.3 as input, we had to settle on a sample size for our multiple regression. We used the harmonic mean[16] because it had a few helpful properties (Jay Verkuilen, personal communication, May 2024). One property is that the sample size is not pulled upward by the largest sample in the group. The sample size we considered is smaller and more conservative than the arithmetic or geometric mean of the sample sizes. The harmonic mean has the advantage of being the natural combination of group sizes when the sizes are uneven.

The results of the regression analysis are shown in Table 2.4. As we expected, burnout at Time 1 was the strongest predictor of burnout at Time 2. The standardized regression weight indicates that for every standard deviation increase in burnout at Time 1, burnout at Time 2 would increase, on average, almost six-tenths of a standard deviation, a large, statistically significant effect. Neither Time-1 resources nor

---

15 This is an example of a concept in statistics called an "ecological" relationship, which, despite its name, does not apply to the branch of biology known as ecology. It refers to relations found in grouped data. Suffice it to say here that the magnitudes of the relationships Lesener et al. found in their structural regression do not necessarily mirror the magnitudes of the relationships among the research participants in the primary studies and are probably overestimates (cf. Robinson, 1950). Schonfeld and Chang (2017) gave an example of an ecological relationship. It involved the correlation, in any given year, between the unemployment rates in the 50 U.S. states and rates of admission to psychiatric hospitals in the states. The correlation between the state level unemployment rate and state level hospitalization rate does not translate to the correlation, among U.S. adults, between job loss and getting hospitalized for a psychiatric disorder. Chances are that the correlation among U.S. workers is far weaker than the relationship found at the state level.

16 Harmonic mean $= n/(1/x_1 + 1/x_2 + 1/x_3 + \ldots + 1/x_n)$, where n is the number of samples, x_1 is the size of the first sample, x_2 is the size of the second sample, and so on. For example, if there were three samples of sizes 4, 7, and 11, the harmonic mean would equal 6.20.

Table 2.4 Predicting burnout at Time 2 using a regression analysis adapted from Lesener et al. (2019) correlations, which are shown in Table 2.3.

Predictors	Regression weight	Standard error	p
Burnout Time 1	.583	.164	.001
Job Resources Time 1	−.072	.153	.641

Time-1 demands were a statistically significant predictor of Time-2 burnout.[17] In a check on the foregoing analysis, Jay Verkuilen, our colleague at the CUNY Graduate Center, created for us a synthetic data set that had the same correlations found in Table 2.3. We used the synthetic data set to replicate the regression and obtained the same results. The structural equation models that Lesener et al. developed, particularly those diagrammed in Figures 4 and 5 of their paper, showed slightly stronger effects for Time-1 demands and resources on Time-2 burnout than the null effects we found. Together their findings and ours underline the modest relationship between working conditions and burnout.

We can't stress enough that readers should keep in mind that the analyses apply to the aggregate level and do not necessarily reflect what was taking place at the level of the individuals who participated in the primary studies in the meta-analysis. Because relationships at the aggregate level are likely stronger than the individual-level relationships, the evidence from the study by Lesener et al. and our own reanalysis suggests that job conditions have at most a small effect on burnout.[18]

---

17 We conducted the regression analysis in stages. In stage 1, we only predicted burnout at Time 2 from burnout at Time 1. The adjusted R-squared was. .403, that is, burnout at Time 1 predicted 40% of the variability of burnout at Time 2, a sizable effect. When we added demands and resources in a second stage, they failed to explain additional variance in burnout at Time 2.
18 In other regression analyses, not shown here, we predicted later (Time-2) job demands and job resources. In each case we used three predictors, earlier (Time-1) demands, resources, and burnout. We found that the best, and only, significant predictor of job demands at Time 2 was Time-1 demands. The best, and only, significant predictor of resources at Time 2 was Time-1 resources.

Guthier et al. (2020)

In a more elaborate meta-analysis, Guthier et al., using longitudinal data from 48 primary studies, also examined the relation of Time-1 job stressors to Time-2 burnout (stressor-effects) and Time-1 burnout to Time-2 job stressors (strain-effects). Unlike Aronsson et al. (2017) and Lesener et al. (2019), Guthier et al. (2020) controlled for the time intervals between the studies' data-collection points, which could help in accounting for heterogeneity in the effect sizes ordinarily found in meta-analyses. Guthier et al., like Lesener et al., organized their meta-analysis around the JD–R model.

The research team, however, recognized that any number of theories of occupational stress, not just the JD–R model, would hold that job stressors would predict later strains like burnout. But only two competing hypotheses have something to say about strain-effects. One, the *drift hypothesis*, suggests that individuals who are affected by strain, for example, by high levels of burnout symptoms at the Time-1 baseline, get transferred or otherwise drift downward by way of social selection processes into worse positions with concomitantly greater exposures to job stressors. By contrast, the *refuge hypothesis* involves upward selection or coping. According to this hypothesis, individuals experiencing high levels of strain will seek out opportunities in the same organization or in another organization such that the new opportunities would come with fewer and/or less intense job stressors. According to the refuge hypothesis, individuals experiencing high symptom levels will later be exposed to lower levels of job stressors.

Guthier et al. also elaborated two hypotheses related to the drift hypothesis. One, the *stressor creation hypothesis*, suggests that exhausted workers, because they have difficulty managing job tasks, experience increased exposure to job stressors (e.g., higher workloads). By contrast, the *stressor perception hypothesis* holds that exhausted workers perceive more job stressors (even if stressors such as the size of the workload do not change). While this hypothesis pertains to perceived stressors, the stressor creation hypothesis underlines the creation of "objective" stressors.

Having averaged regression coefficients from the primary longitudinal studies, Guthier et al. found that the average effect of job stressors on burnout[19] (the stressor-effect) was smaller than the average effect of burnout on job stressors (the strain-effect). Because of the way they conducted the research, the findings of Guthier et al. better apply to the individual level than the results of the regression in the meta-analysis by Lesener et al. and our reanalysis of Lesener et al.'s results. As per the JD–R model, Guthier et al. evaluated the extent to which job control and job support, as reflected in country-level data from the 2010 European Working Conditions Survey (Eurofund, 2012), buffered or mitigated the impact of job stressors on burnout (the stressor-effect) and burnout on stressors (the strain-effect). These findings indicated that increased job control or job support reduced the influence of Time-1 burnout on Time-2 job stressors (the strain-effect), but neither job control nor job support modified the impact of job stressors on later burnout (the stressor-effect). We note that Guthier et al. evaluated the buffering effect of the resources job control and job support using *aggregated* country-level job data. However, the country-level job control and job support factors do not necessarily reflect job resources at the participant level. The meta-analysis did not or could not include those kinds of participant-level resources because the relevant measures or interaction terms were absent from the primary studies.

A close look at the analyses revealed that the modest effect of job stressors on later (emotional) exhaustion (stressor effect, $\beta = .0062$) was statistically significant. By contrast, the impact of exhaustion on later job stressors was significant ($\beta = .0123$) and *larger than* the stressor-effect. Guthier et al.'s findings were strikingly consistent with Schaufeli and Enzmann's (1998) conclusions from more than 20 years earlier regarding the modest impact of job stressors on burnout. Regarding depersonalization/cynicism, neither the stressor-effect nor the strain-effect was significant. These findings underline the centrality of exhaustion in burnout. Guthier et al. did not examine reduced personal accomplishment "because it is unclear if it represents a component or an outcome of burnout and because the vast majority of studies did not assess it" (p. 1147).

---

19 If a primary study assessed both exhaustion and depersonalization/cynicism, Guthier et al. used an overall burnout score; however, if only one score was assessed, e.g., exhaustion, that score was used to represent burnout (C. Guthier and C. Dormann, personal communications, September 2024).

Guthier et al. (2020) evaluated potential publication bias. They found bigger stressor effects in small-sample studies than in large-sample studies, suggesting publication bias. The researchers, however, found that sample size was not related to strain-effects of burnout on job stressors.

Other methodological issues emerged. The researchers found differences in the size of stressor-effects when comparing studies that hypothesized such effects and studies that did not. Unlike studies in which stressor-effects on burnout were hypothesized, studies that did *not* hypothesize stressor-effects revealed statistically significant *negative* effects, suggesting a bias known in the research community as HARKing, an acronym for Hypothesizing After the Results are Known. Moreover, in studies that did not hypothesize a strain-effect of burnout on job stressors, the effect of burnout on job stressors was significant. By contrast, in studies that did hypothesize a strain-effect of burnout on job stressors, the strain-effect was lower. These latter results also suggest HARKing bias. Guthier et al.'s statistical power analyses suggested that studies that detected an effect of job stressors on burnout mainly reflected chance findings.

Given the more solid results bearing on the strain-effect of burnout leading to increased exposure to job stressors, the findings are more compatible with the drift hypothesis than the refuge hypothesis (which predicts that strains lead to reduced exposure to job stressors). Neither the stressor-creation hypothesis nor the stressor-perception hypothesis could be ruled out. In other words, it could not be determined if workers with higher levels of burnout symptoms objectively go on to encounter more job stressors or perceive more job stressors. However, because stressors at baseline were statistically controlled, we give more weight to the stressor-creation hypothesis.

Summary of the Meta-analyses' Findings

Two problems with Aronsson et al.'s (2017) meta-analysis limit the light it can shed on the magnitude of stressor-effects. First, they mixed together better controlled longitudinal studies with case-control studies. Second, they employed a diagnosis-like version of burnout as their dependent variable, which is problematic given burnout's diagnostic heterogeneity. In addition, they did not test for a reverse-causal strain-effect hypothesis.

The meta-analyses by Lesener et al. (2019) and Guthier et al. (2020) suggest that job stressors do exert effects on burnout but that these effects are modest. Factors such as job demands were based on self-reports. However, by controlling for Time-1 burnout in evaluating the influence of Time-1 job demands on later burnout, there was a degree of statistical control for symptom levels biasing the reporting of baseline demands. The results of these meta-analyses are consistent with conclusions drawn many years earlier. Schaufeli (2003) concluded that "when a rigorous selection is made of longitudinal studies that assess the effects of antecedents on *changes* in burnout levels, virtually no causal effects are found" (p. 8). By antecedents, Schaufeli referred to workplace stressors such as work overload. He went on to observe that because burnout symptoms are highly stable, there was little space for baseline workplace stressors to affect later symptoms.

Conclusions

In their early publications, Freudenberger and Maslach, in making the concept of burnout known to the research community and the public, underlined the impact of interactional stressors on helping professionals. Later the burnout concept was applied to a wider variety of occupations. Freudenberger and Maslach regarded work-related psychological or emotional exhaustion as the core of burnout. According to Maslach, however, there are two other burnout-related dimensions, depersonalization/cynicism and reduced personal accomplishment/inefficacy. Those latter feelings are assumed to result from job-related exhaustion. Emotional exhaustion, depersonalization, and reduced accomplishment are embodied in the original MBI, which was published in 1981, and in later variants of the original instrument. The dimensions of burnout, however, appear to have been predefined, having already been described in data-free articles published between 1976 and 1978. In the papers that laid the foundation of the concept of burnout, a surprising lacuna stands out. References to previously published and contemporaneous research on the impact of life stressors and job stressors on mental and physical health were absent.

Fifty years after the first papers on burnout were published, fierce debates continue to surround the most basic aspects of burnout's definition

(Bianchi & Schonfeld, 2024a,b). The widely endorsed view that burnout is a syndrome comprising exhaustion, depersonalization/cynicism, and reduced accomplishment/inefficacy has a shaky foundation and continues to raise serious concerns. The three "components" of burnout lack cohesiveness and do not cover the symptoms exhibited by stressed-out workers as described in Chapter 1. Many of the claims that accompanied the introduction of the burnout construct were evidence-free and remain ill-supported. Burnout has some relation to occupational stressors, but the most advanced meta-analysis to date (Guthier et al., 2020) suggests that it is more predictive of the later occurrence of job stressors than it is a result of exposure to job stressors. Notwithstanding sensationalist communication on an ongoing burnout pandemic (cf. Schonfeld & Bianchi, 2021), the prevalence of the syndrome is, in fact, unknown because of the absence of sound, consensual diagnostic criteria for the condition. Although the MBI has been regarded as the gold standard for assessing burnout, the psychometric (e.g., the patina of reliability) and structural properties of the instrument have proven to be problematic (e.g., in terms of syndromal unity and discriminant validity).

That the MBI does *not* produce a burnout score counts among the oddities of burnout research (Bianchi et al., 2024). Given the importance of the burnout construct in occupational health research and practice, the pervasive problems that affect the construct are disquieting. Shirom (2005) already raised the difficult question of whether burnout constitutes a "real phenomenon," existing "apart from the awareness and interpretation of the individual researcher" (see also Friberg, 2009). In the next chapter, we delve into the issue of the distinctiveness of the burnout syndrome vis-à-vis depressive conditions and, by implication, the (discriminant) validity of the burnout construct.

References

Alvarez, K. P. (2015). *The Stanford Prison Experiment*. Sandbar Pictures and Abandon Pictures.
American Psychiatric Association. (2013). *Diagnostic and statistical manual of mental disorders* (5th ed.). American Psychiatric Publishing.
Anastasi, A., & Urbina, S. (1997). *Psychological testing* (7th ed.). Prentice-Hall.

Aronsson, G., Theorell, T., Grape, T., Hammarström, A., Hogstedt, C., Marteinsdottir, I., Skoog, I., Träskman-Bendz, L., & Hall, C. (2017). A systematic review including meta-analysis of work environment and burnout symptoms. *BMC Public Health*, *17*(1), 264. https://doi.org/10.1186/s12889-017-4153-7

Bakker, A. B., Schaufeli, W. B., Demerouti, E., Janssen, P. P. M., Van Der Hulst, R., & Brouwer, J. (2000). Using equity theory to examine the difference between burnout and depression. *Anxiety, Stress, & Coping*, *13*(3), 247-268. https://doi.org/10.1080/10615800008549265

Bianchi, R., & Schonfeld, I. S. (2023). Examining the evidence base for burnout. *Bulletin of the World Health Organization*, *101*, 743-745. http://dx.doi.org/10.2471/BLT.23.289996

Bianchi, R., & Schonfeld, I. S. (2024a). Burnout: Half a century of controversy. *Occupational Medicine*, *74*(6), 400-402. htps://doi.org/10.1093/occmed/kqae052

Bianchi, R., & Schonfeld, I. S. (2024b). Beliefs about burnout. *Work & Stress*. htps://doi.org/10.1080/02678373.2024.2364590

Bianchi, R., Swingler, G., & Schonfeld, I. S. (2024). The Maslach Burnout Inventory is not a measure of burnout. *WORK: A Journal of Prevention, Assessment & Rehabilitation*, *79*(3), 1525-1527. https://doi.org/10.3233/WOR-240095

Bianchi, R., Verkuilen, J., Sowden, J. F., & Schonfeld, I. S. (2023). Toward a new approach to job-related distress: A three-sample study of the Occupational Depression Inventory. *Stress & Health*, *39*(1), 137-153. https://doi.org/10.1002/smi.3177

Bianchi, R., Verkuilen, J., Toker, S., Schonfeld, I. S., Gerber, M., Brähler, E., & Kroenke, K. (2022). Is the PHQ-9 a unidimensional measure of depression? A 58,272-participant study. *Psychological Assessment*, *34*(6), 595-603. https://doi.org/10.1037/pas0001124

Borenstein, M., Hedges, L. V., Higgins, J. P. T., & Rothstein, H. (2021). *Introduction to meta-analysis* (2nd ed.). John Wiley & Sons.

Bradley, H. B. (1969). Community-based treatment for young adult offenders. *Crime & Delinquency*, *15*(3), 359-370. https://doi.org/10.1177/001112876901500307

Brown, G. W., Harris, T. O., & Peto, J. (1973). Life events and psychiatric disorders. 2. Nature of causal link. *Psychological Medicine*, *3*(2), 159-176. https://doi.org/10.1017/s0033291700048492

Burr, H., Berthelsen, H., Moncada, S., Nübling, M., Dupret, E., Demiral, Y., Oudyk, J., Kristensen, T. S., Llorens, C., Navarro, A., Lincke, H.-J., Bocéréan, C., Sahan, C., Smith, P., & Pohrt, A. (2019). The third version of the Copenhagen Psychosocial Questionnaire. *Safety and Health at Work, 10*(4), 482–503. https://doi.org/10.1016/j.shaw.2019.10.002

Campbell, D. T., & Fiske, D. W. (1959). Convergent and discriminant validation by the multitrait–multimethod matrix. *Psychological Bulletin, 56*(2), 81–105. https://doi.org/10.1037/h0046016

Canter, M. B., & Freudenberger, L. (2001). Obituary: Herbert J Freudenberger (1926–1999). *American Psychologist, 56*(12), 1171. https://doi.org/10.1037/0003-066X.56.12.1171

Caplan, R. D., Cobb, S., French, J. R. P., Jr., Harrison, R. V., & Pinneau, S. R., Jr. (1975). *Job demands and worker health: Main effects and occupational differences* (U.S. Department of Health, Education, and Welfare, Publication No. [NIOSH] 75-160). U.S. Government Printing Office. [Also published by the Institute for Social Research, University of Michigan, 1980.]

Cohen, J. (1977). *Statistical power analysis for the behavioral sciences*. Lawrence Erlbaum.

Cohen, J., Cohen, P., West, S. G., & Aiken, L. S. (2003). *Applied multiple regression/correlation analysis for the behavioral sciences*, (3rd ed.). Lawrence Erlbaum Associates Publishers.

COPSOQ International Network. (2024, May 8, 2024). *Publications on COPSOQ*. https://www.copsoq-network.org/publications-on-copsoq/

Demerouti, E., Bakker, A. B., Nachreiner, F., & Schaufeli, W. B. (2001). The job demands–resources model of burnout. *Journal of Applied Psychology, 86*(3), 499–512. https://doi.org/10.1037/0021-9010.86.3.499

Dohrenwend, B. S. (1973). Social status and stressful life events. *Journal of Personality and Social Psychology, 28*(2), 225–235. https://doi.org/10.1037/h0035718

Enzmann, D. (2005). Burnout and emotions: An underresearched issue in search of a theory. In A.-S. G. Antoniou & C. L. Cooper (Eds.), *Research Companion to Organizational Health Psychology*. (pp. 495–502). Edward Elgar Publishing. https://doi.org/10.4337/9781845423308.00042

Eurofund. (2012). *Fifth European Working Conditions Survey*. Publications Office of the European Union.

Freudenberger, H. J. (1973). The psychologist in a free clinic setting: An alternative model in health care. *Psychotherapy: Theory, Research and Practice, 10*(1), 52–61. https://doi.org/10.1037/h0087545

Freudenberger, H. J. (1974). Staff burnout. *Journal of Social Issues, 30*(1), 159–165. https://doi.org/10.1111/j.1540-4560.1974.tb00706.x

Freudenberger, H. J. (1975). The staff burnout syndrome in alternative institutions. *Psychotherapy: Theory, Research, and Practice, 12*(1), 72–83. https://doi.org/10.1037/h0086411

Friberg, R. (2009). Burnout: From popular culture to psychiatric diagnosis in Sweden. *Culture, Medicine, and Psychiatry, 33*(4), 538–558. https://doi.org/10.1007/s11013-009-9149-z

Friedman, M., Rosenman, R. H., & Carroll, V. (1958). Changes in the serum cholesterol and blood clotting time in men subjected to cyclic variation of occupational stress. *Circulation, 17*, 852–861. https://doi.org/10.1161/01.CIR.17.5.852

Ginsburg, S. G. (1974). The problem of the burned out executive. *Personnel Journal, 48*(8), 598–600.

Gold medal award for life achievement in the practice of psychology: Herbert J Freudenberger. (1999). *American Psychologist, 54*(8), 578–580. https://doi.org/10.1037/h0090473

Goldberg, D. P. (1972). *The detection of psychiatric illness by questionnaire: A technique for the identification and assessment of non-psychotic psychiatric illness.* Oxford University Press.

Greene, G. (1961). *A burnt-out case.* The Viking Press.

Guthier, C., Dormann, C., & Voelkle, M. C. (2020). Reciprocal effects between job stressors and burnout: A continuous time meta-analysis of longitudinal studies. *Psychological Bulletin, 146*(12), 1146–1173. https://doi.org/10.1037/bul0000304

Hathaway, S. R., & McKinley, J. C. (1940). A multiphasic personality schedule (Minnesota): I. Construction of the schedule. *Journal of Psychology, 10*, 249–254. https://doi.org/10.1080/00223980.1940.9917000

Hobfoll, S. E. (1989). Conservation of resources: A new attempt at conceptualizing stress. *American Psychologist, 44*(3), 513–524. https://doi.org/10.1037/0003-066X.44.3.513

Hobfoll, S. E., & Shirom, A. (2001). Conservation of resources theory: Applications to stress and management in the workplace. In R. T. Golembiewski (Ed.), *Handbook of Organizational Behavior* (2nd ed., pp. 57–80). Marcel Dekker.

Kahn, R. L., Wolfe, D. M., Quinn, R. P., Snoek, J., & Rosenthal, R. A. (1964). *Organizational stress: Studies in role conflict and ambiguity.* Wiley.

Kobasa, S. C. (1979). Stressful life events, personality, and health: Inquiry into hardiness. *Journal of Personality and Social Psychology, 37*(1), 1–11. https://doi.org/10.1037/0022-3514.37

Kristensen, T. S., Borritz, M., Villadsen, E., & Christensen, K. B. (2005a). The Copenhagen Burnout Inventory: A new tool for the assessment of burnout. *Work & Stress, 19*(3), 192–207. https://doi.org/10.1080/02678370500297720

Kristensen, T. S., Hannerz, H., Hogh, A. & Borg, V. (2005b). The Copenhagen Psychosocial Questionnaire—a tool for the assessment and improvement of the psychosocial work environment. *Scandinavian Journal of Work, Environment & Health, 31*(6), 438–449. https://doi.org/10.5271/sjweh.948

Kristensen, T. S. (2010). A questionnaire is more than a questionnaire. *Scandinavian Journal of Public Health, 38*(3 Suppl), 149–155. https://doi.org/10.1177/1403494809354437

Langner, T. S. (1962). A twenty-two item screening score of psychiatric symptoms as indicating impairment. *Journal of Health and Human Behavior, 3*(4), 269–276. https://doi.org/10.2307/2948599

Le Texier, T. (2019). Debunking the Stanford prison experiment. *American Psychologist, 74*(7), 823–839. https://doi.org/10.1037/amp0000401

Leiter, M. P., & Durup, J. (1994). The discriminant validity of burnout and depression: A confirmatory factor analytic study. *Anxiety, Stress, and Coping, 7*, 357–373. http://dx.doi.org/10.1080/10615809408249357

Lesener, T., Gusy, B., & Wolter, C. (2019). The job demands-resources model: A meta-analytic review of longitudinal studies. *Work & Stress, 33*(1), 76–103. https://doi.org/10.1080/02678373.2018.1529065

Martin, D. (1999, Dec. 5). Herbert Freudenberger, 73, coiner of 'burnout,' is dead. *The New York Times*.

Maslach, C. (1976, Sept.). Burned-out. *Human Behavior: The Newsmagazine of the Social Science, 5*(9), 16–22.

Maslach, C. (1978). The client role in staff burn-out. *Journal of Social Issues, 34*(4), 111–124. https://doi.org/10.1111/j.1540-4560.1978.tb00778.x

Maslach, C. (1993). Burnout: A multidimensional perspective. In W. B. Schaufeli, C. Maslach, & T. Marek (Eds.), *Professional burnout: Recent developments in theory and research* (pp. 19–32). Taylor & Francis.

Maslach, C., & Jackson, S. E. (1981). The measurement of experienced burnout. *Journal of Organizational Behavior, 2*(2), 99–113. https://doi.org/10.1002/job.4030020205

Maslach, C., Jackson, S. E., & Leiter, M. P. (1996). *Maslach Burnout Inventory manual* (3rd ed.). Consulting Psychologists Press.

Maslach, C., Jackson, S. E., & Leiter, M. P. (2016). *Maslach Burnout Inventory manual* (4th ed.). Consulting Psychologists Press.

Maslach, C., & Leiter, M. (1997). *The truth about burnout: How organizations cause personal stress and what to do about it*. Jossey-Bass.

Maslach, C., & Pines, A. (1977). The burn-out syndrome in the day care setting. *Child Youth Care Forum, 6*(2), 100–113.

Maslach, C., & Schaufeli, W. B. (1993). Historical and conceptual development of burnout. In W. B. Schaufeli, C. Maslach, & T. Marek (Eds.), *Professional burnout: Recent developments in theory and research* (pp. 2–18). Taylor & Francis.

Maslach, C., Schaufeli, W. B., & Leiter, M. P. (2001). Job burnout. *Annual Review of Psychology, 52* (1), 397–422. https://doi.org/10.1146/annurev.psych.52.1.397

Meier, S. T. (1984). The construct validity of burnout. *Journal of Occupational Psychology, 53*(3), 211–219. https://doi.org/10.1111/j.2044-8325.1984.tb00163.x

Pines, A., Aronson, E., & Kalfry, D. (1981). *Burnout: From tedium to personal growth*. The Free Press.

Pines, A., & Maslach, C. (1978). Characteristics of staff burnout in mental health settings. *Hospital & Community Psychiatry, 29*(4), 233–237. https://doi.org/10.1176/ps.29.4.233

Radloff, L. S. (1977). The CES-D Scale: A self-report depression scale for research in the general population. *Applied Psychological Measurement, 1*(3), 384–401. https://doi.org/10.1177/014662167700100306

Robinson, W. S. (1950). Ecological correlations and the behavior of individuals. *American Sociological Review, 15*(3), 352–357. http://dx.doi.org/10.2307/2087176

Rotenstein, L. S., Torre, M., Ramos, M. A., Rosales, R. C., Guille, C., Sen, S., & Mata, D. A. (2018). Prevalence of burnout among physicians: A systematic review. *Journal of the American Medical Association, 320*(11), 1131–1150. https://doi.org/10.1001/jama.2018.12777

Schaufeli, W. B. (2003). Past performance and future perspectives of burnout research. *SA Journal of Industrial Psychology, 29*(4), 1–15. https://hdl.handle.net/10520/EJC88982

Schaufeli, W. B., & Enzmann, D. (1998). *The burnout companion to study and practice: A critical analysis*. Taylor & Francis.

Schaufeli, W. B., Leiter, M. P., Maslach, C. (2009). Burnout: 35 years of research and practice. *Career Development International, 14*(3), 304–320. https://doi.org/10.1108/13620430910966406

Schonfeld, I. S., & Bianchi, R. (2021). Psychiatrist burnout. *American Journal of Psychiatry, 178*(2), 204. https://doi.org/10.1176/appi.ajp.2020.20071110

Schonfeld, I. S., & Chang, C.-H. (2017). *Occupational health psychology: Work, stress, and health.* Springer Publishing Company. https://doi.org/10.1891/9780826199683

Schonfeld, I. S., & Feinman, S. J. (2012). Difficulties of alternatively certified teachers. *Education and Urban Society, 44*(3), 215–246. https://doi.org/10.1177/0013124510392570

Schonfeld, I. S., & Mazzola, J.J. (2013). Strengths and limitations of qualitative approaches to research in occupational health psychology. In R. Sinclair, M. Wang, & L. Tetrick (Eds.), *Research Methods in Occupational Health Psychology: State of the Art in Measurement, Design, and Data Analysis* (pp. 268–289). Routledge. https://doi.org/10.4324/9780203095249

Schonfeld, I. S., Verkuilen, J., & Bianchi, R. (2019). Inquiry into the correlation between burnout and depression. *Journal of Occupational Health Psychology, 24,* 603–616. http://dx.doi.org/10.1037/ocp0000151

Selye, H. (1956). *The stress of life.* McGraw-Hill.

Shirom, A. (2005). Reflections on the study of burnout. *Work & Stress, 19*(3), 263–270. https://doi.org/10.1080/02678370500376649

Shirom, A., & Melamed, S. (2006). A comparison of the construct validity of two burnout measures in two groups of professionals. *International Journal of Stress Management, 13*(2), 176–200. https://doi.org/10.1037/1072-5245.13.2.176

Sommer, R. (1973). The burnt-out chairman. *American Psychologist, 28*(6), 536–537. https://doi.org/10.1037/h0038106

World Health Organization. (2022). *International statistical classification of diseases and related health problems* (11th ed.). Author.

Zahneis, M. (2018, Sept. 21). How a decades-old experiment sparked a war over the future of psychology. *Chronicle of Higher Education.* https://www.chronicle.com/article/how-a-decades-old-experiment-sparked-a-war-over-the-future-of-psychology/s

3

Burnout–Depression Overlap

What is the basis for distinguishing burnout from depression? Is there a clear reason to assume burnout to be a nondepressive condition? Many attempts at distinguishing burnout from depression have been troubling. Melnick et al. (2017), for example, compared burnout, considered dimensionally, to depression, considered diagnostically or categorically. Such a comparison reduces depression to its clinical stage, focusing only on the high end of the continuum of depression (at which a disorder can be formally diagnosed), while approaching burnout as a continuous factor. The comparison, which truncates depression, is methodologically problematic, reducing the magnitude of the burnout–depression correlation.[1] To express this idea in the vernacular of a blackjack player, correlating burnout as a dimension and depression as a present-or-absent diagnosis stacks the deck against finding a high correlation. A more appropriate approach to burnout–depression overlap involves considering both variables dimensionally and examining both continua in their entirety. As described later in this chapter, various analytical techniques, including factor analysis, have allowed researchers to examine burnout and depression as continua. Another approach would involve comparing individuals at the high and low ends of the depression continuum to individuals at the high and low ends of the burnout continuum.

---

1 In this example, the full spectrum of scores on a depressive symptom scale is reduced to a binary factor representing depression-present or depression-absent. As shown in Chapter 1, a great deal of information is lost, and the size of the burnout–depression correlation is thereby reduced.

Breaking Point: Job Stress, Occupational Depression, and the Myth of Burnout, First Edition. Irvin Sam Schonfeld and Renzo Bianchi.
© 2025 John Wiley & Sons, Inc. Published 2025 by John Wiley & Sons, Inc.

Perhaps the main constituent of the argument in support of the burnout–depression distinction has been the job-relatedness ascribed to burnout (e.g., Maslach et al., 2001). According to this argument, burnout is a job-specific, work-induced condition whereas depression is a general, "context-free" condition. Schaufeli et al. (2009) suggested that there is something inherently job-related about burnout:

> a multi-dimensional approach as in the MBI is by definition incompatible with the notion of context-free burnout. Then in any context—at work or outside work—people may feel exhausted, but cynicism and reduced professional efficacy refer to a particular object (i.e., one is cynical about something and feels inefficacious to do something). A retired or unemployed person may feel exhausted, but it is impossible to identify the "something" about which unemployed or retired people should feel cynical or inefficacious. (p. 212)

The job-relatedness argument has proven to be problematic for several reasons. First, the attempt to essentialize the relationship between burnout and the job falls short. One may also feel cynical toward other aspects of one's life (e.g., one's marriage) and inefficacious in the context of other roles (e.g., parenting). Second, the job-related character of a condition does not change the fundamental nature of that condition. For example, job-related anxiety and depressive symptoms remain anxiety and depressive symptoms. Job-related back pain remains back pain. A cancer caused by chemical exposures in the workplace remains cancer. In other words, burnout could be viewed as job-related *and* depressive in nature without the slightest contradiction. Third, consistent with the meta-analytic findings of Guthier et al. (2020), spotlighted in Chapter 2, burnout may not be as job-related as generally assumed. There is, in fact, little evidence that burnout is primarily or specifically predicted by job stressors. While job stressors predict burnout, the association appears to be small and leaves most of the variance in burnout unexplained. Notwithstanding the narratives that surround burnout, its etiology is far from having been elucidated. Conclusive evidence that, compared to depression, burnout is more strongly caused by job-related factors remains to be produced. It is worth bearing in mind that Maslach took the causal link between job stressors and burnout for granted as early as 1976, at a time when not a single scientific study of burnout's etiology had been published and burnout was not defined with any degree of clarity.

The Idea of a Syndrome

Far and away, the MBI has been the most commonly used instrument to assess burnout, and the most common definition of burnout derives from the MBI (Schaufeli et al., 2009; Schonfeld et al., 2019a). Even the World Health Organization's tripartite definition of burnout is based on the MBI (Bianchi & Schonfeld, 2023).

Burnout, as per the MBI, is supposed to be a syndrome. To reiterate what we wrote in Chapter 2, according to the *DSM-5* (American Psychiatric Association [APA], 2013), a syndrome is a "grouping of signs and symptoms, based on their frequent co-occurrence." Given the idea of "frequent co-occurrence," we encapsulated Maslach et al.'s (2001) tripartite conception of burnout in a Popperian[2] "syndromal hypothesis" (Bianchi et al., 2021; Schonfeld & Bianchi, 2021a, b). According to that hypothesis, the three symptoms of burnout, emotional exhaustion (EE; which has also been called just exhaustion), depersonalization (DP; also called cynicism), and reduced personal accomplishment (PA, also called professional inefficacy), should be more closely related to each other than to symptoms that are not part of the syndrome, for example, depressive symptoms. We also note that EE is burnout's core dimension (Maslach et al., 2001).

First Look at Burnout-Depression Overlap

When comparing burnout with depression, unresolvable stress immediately appears as a common etiological denominator. Job stressors, for example, contribute to the development of both burnout and depressive symptoms.

---

2 See Chapter 1 on Karl Popper on the importance of hypotheses.

The idea of burnout–depression overlap, however, begins with the very first paper *exclusively* devoted to burnout and published in a social science journal.[3] That paper, written by Herbert J. Freudenberger and published in 1974 in the *Journal of Social Issues*, was entitled "Staff Burn-Out." Freudenberger identified symptoms and signs of burnout to include irritability, being easily frustrated and angered, fatigue, and inflexibility. He wrote that the burned-out person "looks, acts and seems depressed" (p. 161).

Relevant to the idea of burnout–depression overlap is the publication in 1981 of a book by Ayala Pines and her colleagues. The book introduced a 21-item scale that later became known as the Burnout Measure (Pines & Aronson, 1988). The scale included items such as "Feeling depressed" and "Feeling hopeless," items that explicitly reflect depressive symptomatology. There was even an anxiety item, "Feeling anxious." The scale, as expected, included items that reflect exhaustion such as "Being physically exhausted" and "Being emotionally exhausted." Pines had previously worked with Maslach. In the late 1970s, the two investigators together conducted some of the first research on burnout.

In 1984, Scott T. Meier, employing a sample of U.S. college faculty, found that the MBI correlated with depressive symptom scales about as strongly as it correlated with two other burnout scales despite the MBI and the depressive symptom scales having different response formats.[4] Meier treated the MBI as one big scale; this was before researchers began to take a more granular approach by looking at the relation of each of the MBI's subscales to depressive symptoms. Future research would single out the central component of the MBI, the exhaustion subscale, for overlap with what depressive-symptom scales measure.

Burnout and Depression as Distinct Constructs

When research on burnout began to accelerate, some psychologists conducted studies of the *construct validity* of burnout scales. The foundation of research in psychology and psychiatry is measurement.

---

3 In Chapter 2, we note that Freudenberger published a paper that briefly touched on burnout one year earlier.
4 Format differences in scales tend to weaken the correlation between scale scores.

If the measures we use do not adequately reflect the constructs psychologists and psychiatrists want to study, whether depression, anxiety, intelligence, school achievement, or others, their research findings will be weak and inconclusive. As mentioned in Chapter 2, construct validity is often demonstrated by showing evidence for a scale's convergent and discriminant validity (Campbell & Fiske, 1959). In a nutshell, the purpose of research on the *convergent validity* of a psychological scale is to show that the scale purported to assess a construct and alternate measures of the same construct are highly correlated. Otherwise, we would question the soundness of the scale. For example, different measures of burnout should be highly correlated with each other. In his study of college faculty, Meier (1984) showed, by virtue of the high correlation of the MBI with two other measures of burnout, that the MBI demonstrated good convergent validity.

A demonstration of construct validity, however, requires more than evidence of convergent validity. It also requires evidence of *discriminant validity* (Rönkkö & Cho, 2022; Spector, 2013). As we mentioned in Chapter 2, discriminant validity underlines construct distinctiveness. It refers to evidence showing that, compared to a scale's correlation with measures of the same construct, the scale's correlation with measures of a theoretically different construct should be much lower. For example, compared to a burnout scale's correlation to other burnout scales, the burnout scale in question should have a much lower correlation with a measure of depression, assuming depression represents a different construct. Meier (1984) found weak evidence for the discriminant validity of the study's three burnout scales. One of the burnout scales in the study was more highly correlated with the short form of the Minnesota Multiphasic Personality Inventory–Depression Scale than with the other two burnout measures. Of course, the discriminant validity of burnout scales goes hand-in-hand with the syndromal hypothesis.

In Chapter 2 we described foundational studies conducted by Leiter and Durup (1994) and Bakker et al. (2000) that claimed to demonstrate the discriminant validity of the MBI. Leiter and Durup, when controlling for measurement error, found an unexpectedly high correlation between burnout and depression factors, $r = .72$. Bakker et al. (2000), after breaking up the Center for Epidemiological Studies Depression scale (CESD) into smaller, less reliable subscales, still found that the correlations between EE and the truncated depressive symptom scales ($r = .68$ and $.56$) were higher than correlations between the EE and DP ($r = .47$) and EE and PA ($r = -.42$).

A Line of Research by Bianchi, Schonfeld, and Colleagues

The authors began their line of research on burnout and depression by studying schoolteachers. Teachers are an apt group to study because the conditions in which they work are highly variable (Schonfeld & Farrell, 2010; Schonfeld & Santiago, 1994). Some teachers work in well-run schools, where they accomplish a great deal and feel safe. Others work in schools that are poorly run, where students are disrespectful, and where teachers are exposed to violence or its threat (Schonfeld, 2006; Schonfeld et al., 2017). Other teachers work in schools that are in-between those poles (Schonfeld, 2000). Because there is so much variability in the quality of the schools in which teachers work, there is likely to be variability in teachers' psychological well-being, given that teachers' well-being is at least partly a function of their working conditions. That variability makes for an appropriate context in which to study the relation between burnout and depression.

The stimulus for the authors' collaboration, as described in the Preface, was Bianchi et al.'s (2013) study of more than 1,600 French schoolteachers. The research team found that the correlation of burnout's core symptom dimension, EE, and the Beck[5] Depression Inventory (BDI-II, i.e., the second edition of the instrument) was .74. By contrast, the correlations among the MBI subscales, EE, DP, and reduced PA ranged from .47 to .51. In other words, the correlation between EE and depressive symptoms was higher than the correlations among the MBI's subscales, which contradicts the syndromal hypothesis.

The authors' first collaboration (Bianchi et al., 2014), which included Eric Laurent, involved a study of 5,575 French schoolteachers. We found the MBI's EE subscale correlated .72 with scores on the PHQ-9 (a measure of depression; Kroenke et al., 2001), which was greater than the correlations among the three MBI subscales.

---

5 The Beck in question is Aaron T. Beck, who figures in Chapters 1 and 5.

A study conducted by Ahola et al. (2005) influenced our approach to the 5,575-teacher sample (Bianchi et al., 2014). Ahola et al. found that 53% of individuals who had "severe burnout," as assessed by the MBI–General Survey, met criteria for a diagnosis of depression. We looked closely at how Ahola et al. defined severe burnout, noting that they used a cutoff score of 3.5 on a frequency scale that ranges from "Never" (0) to "Every day" (6) over the course of a year.

We considered the 3.5 cutoff used by Ahola et al. to be too liberal in view of (1) Maslach et al.'s (1996) description of burnout as "a crisis in one's relationship with work" and (2) Schaufeli and Buunk's (2004) depiction of burnout as "a final stage in a breakdown in adaptation." Ahola et al.'s (2005) cutoff score of 3.5 is between burnout symptoms occurring between an average of once per month and once a week, not necessarily reflecting a crisis or a personal breakdown. The implication of using such a liberal cutoff to mark a severe condition is that the burnout group would have to include individuals who were false positives. Because there are no consensual diagnostic criteria for burnout (cf. Rotenstein et al., 2018), we regarded burnout, as per Maslach et al. and Schaufeli and Buunk, as reflecting an average score of 5 or more on the symptom items that make up the MBI's 0–6 scale. A score of 5 reflects burnout symptoms being experienced a few times every week over the course of a year.

We created two groups of teachers. The burnout group comprised 67 teachers who scored 5 or more on the MBI. We contrasted that group to a no-burnout group, which consisted of 750 teachers with scores of 1 (burnout symptoms occurring, on average, at most a few times a year) or less. Just as we required a high threshold to exclude false positives from the burnout group, we excluded from the no-burnout group individuals with scores above 1 to minimize the risk of including false negatives. As shown in Table 3.1, the differences between the burnout and no-burnout groups were stark. We found that 90% of the members of the burnout group met criteria for a provisional diagnosis of a major depressive disorder (MDD),[6] but only 3% of the members of the no-burnout group met those criteria. The table also shows that the

---

[6] We did not have the means to administer a diagnostic interview to the teachers to arrive at a more definitive diagnosis. Instead, we arrived on a provisional diagnosis of

Table 3.1 Differences between the burnout group and the no-burnout group.

	Burnout group	No-burnout group	p
Met criteria for a provisional dx for depression	90%	3%	.001
Currently taking antidepressant medication	30%	4%	.001
History of depression	63%	15%	.001
Suicidal thoughts	60%	4%	.001

Adapted from Bianchi et al., (2014).

proportions of members of the burnout group were more likely to be taking antidepressant medication and have a history of depression. Most concerning is that members of the burnout group were considerably more likely to report experiencing at least some suicidal ideation over the two-week period covered by the PHQ-9.

Schonfeld and Bianchi (2016) decided to study burnout in a different way. Rather than use the MBI, we used the 14-item version (Toker et al., 2012) of the Shirom–Melamed Burnout Measure (SMBM; Shirom & Melamed, 2006). The SMBM ratings range from 1 (a symptom occurring "never or almost never") to 7 (a symptom occurring "always or almost always"). We also conducted the research in a different country, the United States, this time with 1,386 schoolteachers. We found the correlation between the total score on the SMBM and the PHQ-9 to be quite high (.77).

We again created two groups. One group, the burnout group, consisted of 124 teachers with SMBM symptom scores that averaged 5.5 or higher, that is to say, teachers who experienced burnout symptoms on average more than "quite frequently." The other group, the no-burnout group, comprised 215 teachers who averaged a score of 2 ("very infrequently) or less on each symptom. We found that 86% of the members of the burnout group met criteria for a provisional diagnosis of depression; however, fewer

---

MDD based on the pattern of responses to the symptom questions on the PHQ-9. The PHQ-9 is keyed to the nine *DSM-5* symptoms of MDD.

than 1% of the members of the no-burnout group met criteria for a provisional diagnosis (see Table 3.2). As shown in the table, members of the burnout group were significantly more likely to have a history of depressive and anxiety disorders and to be taking antidepressant and antianxiety medication. Again, most concerning is that members of the burnout group were much more likely to report experiencing at least some suicidal ideation over the two-week period the PHQ-9 covered.

The authors also began to study the nomological networks of burnout and depression in greater detail (Bianchi & Schonfeld, 2016; Schonfeld & Bianchi, 2016). The term "nomological network" refers to the system of relations, within a theoretical framework, among observable properties and among theoretical constructs (Cronbach & Meehl, 1955). We hypothesized that if burnout reflects depression (as a continuous dimension), then the nomological networks of burnout and depression scales would parallel each other.

We (Schonfeld & Bianchi, 2016) found that the SMBM and the PHQ-9, that is, burnout and depressive symptoms, were similarly related to *stressful life events occurring outside of work*, job adversity, and coworker support. The relationship of the two scales with job adversity was particularly interesting because the SMBM, like other burnout scales, has an advantage in terms of its potential to correlate with job adversity because

Table 3.2 Differences between the burnout group and the no-burnout group.

	Burnout group	No-burnout group	p
Met criteria for a provisional dx for depression	86%	0.5%	.001
Currently taking antidepressant medication	30%	4%	.001
History of depression	37%	13%	.001
Currently taking antidepressant medication	26%	7%	.001
History of anxiety disorder	30%	13%	.001
Currently taking antianxiety medication	14%	6%	.001
Suicidal thoughts	36%	2%	.001

Adapted from Schonfeld & Bianchi, (2016).

the burnout scale explicitly contextualizes the symptoms as having been experienced within the work domain. Both the SMBM and the PHQ-9 correlated with job adversity .30 despite the PHQ-9 not referencing work.

In a paper critical of our research, Maslach and Leiter (2016) claimed that our finding a high correlation between the burnout's exhaustion core and depressive symptoms was an artifact. They argued that depression scales include symptoms of burnout, artificially boosting the correlation. Of course, we could have counter-argued that burnout–depression overlap is caused by burnout scales including symptoms of depression. Depression scales such as the Beck Depression Inventory (Beck et al., 1961), the Center for Epidemiologic Studies—Depression scale (Radloff, 1977), and the Minnesota Multiphasic Personality Inventory's Depression scale (O'Connor et al., 1957) were developed long before burnout scales were introduced. And each scale contains items referencing fatigue and/or sleep problems. Depression is a much older construct than burnout, and psychologists and psychiatrists have long known about feelings of fatigue and sleep problems plaguing individuals who are depressed. Feelings of fatigue and sleep problems are basic aspects of depression.

Together with our colleague Jay Verkuilen (Schonfeld et al., 2019a), we used three samples to evaluate Maslach and Leiter's (2016) criticism. The samples comprised French and U.S. schoolteachers. Two studies used the MBI and one, the SMBM. One of the study's aims was to examine the relation between burnout's exhaustion symptoms and depressive symptoms by excluding depressive symptom items that potentially overlap with burnout (e.g., fatigue and sleep problems).

We used confirmatory factor analysis (CFA) to estimate the correlations among the burnout and depression factors—to be conservative, we deliberately derived the depression factor from symptom items other than the fatigue or sleep problems items—controlling for measurement error. A CFA produces correlations that, to some extent, resemble the disattenuated correlations we discussed in Chapter 2, although a CFA is more complex. We obtained correlations of .88, .83, and .84 between each study's burnout-related exhaustion factor and a depression factor, underlining burnout–depression overlap.[7]

---

[7] The version of the SMBM we used contains a three-item emotional exhaustion subscale; however, we found that only one the subscale's three items unambiguously reflected MBI-like emotional exhaustion. The other two items reflected MBI-like

Bianchi, Schonfeld, and Verkuilen (2020) also applied CFAs to burnout and depression data collected in five French and Swiss samples. Three of the samples comprised educators and two samples, individuals employed in diverse occupations. Burnout was assessed with the SMBM and different versions of the MBI. Latent factors (shorn of measurement error) were derived from the correlations among (sub) scale items. We examined the correlations between depressive symptoms and the burnout subscales in two different ways in each sample. In one way, the depression factor involved all nine PHQ-9 symptom items. In the second way, which we performed for comparative purposes, we removed three PHQ-9 items, the items assessing symptoms of fatigue, sleep disturbance, and impaired concentration.

The Exhaustion factor was closely linked to the Depression factor in every sample. Moreover, correlations changed little when we used the shortened PHQ-9 in creating the Depression factor. In other words, Exhaustion was strongly correlated with the Depression factor, regardless. For example, Depression correlated with Exhaustion .81 in the fourth sample when the entire PHQ-9 was used and .76, when the shortened version was used. In the two samples that used the MBI, the Exhaustion factor was more highly correlated with the Depression factor than with Depersonalization/Cynicism and Personal Accomplishment/Professional Efficacy factors, contradicting the syndromal hypothesis.

Burnout and Depressive Cognition

As part of our exploration of the nomological networks of burnout and depression, we compared the relation of teachers' scores on the burnout and depression scales to a depressive cognitive style

---

depersonalization. Given the dearth of items and lack of construct coherence, it was no surprise that this version of emotional exhaustion correlated with the depression factor only .64, which, in itself, is a high correlation given the context. The depression factor correlated .83 with the SMBM physical fatigue factor. We were very conservative in evaluating the overlap with depression in our study of the SMBM in view of the SMBM's having a cognitive weariness subscale. We, therefore, in addition to omitting the PHQ-9 depressive symptoms sleep problems and fatigue symptom items, also omitted the depressive symptom item, problems concentrating. Nevertheless, the cognitive weariness symptom factor correlated .75 with the depressive symptom factor based on six rather than the nine PHQ items.

(Bianchi & Schonfeld, 2016). Depressive cognitive styles include dysfunctional attitudes (e.g., setting unrealistically high standards for oneself, standards a person is likely to fail to reach), rumination, and pessimism. We found that the burnout scale and the depressive symptom scale were startlingly similar in their relation to all three cognitive style indices. For example, among women teachers, burnout symptoms correlated with pessimism .53, while depression correlated with pessimism .57. We broke down the pessimism scale into subscales, one of which was feelings of helplessness. Helplessness, as described in Chapter 1, is characteristic of depression. We found that in women burnout and depression correlated with helplessness at .50 and .51, respectively. In men, the correlations were almost the same, .55 and .50. The correlations of burnout and depression with all three depressive cognitive styles were of highly similar strength, suggesting that burnout intersects depression in terms of cognitive vulnerabilities.

The idea that burnout is associated with a depressive cognitive style is supported by several studies that focused on how people perform on actual tasks and tests, that is, focused on what people *do* beyond what they may declare. Bianchi and Laurent (2015) conducted an eye-tracking study in which participants were asked to watch a series of slides consisting of emotional and neutral pictures. The gaze of the participants was recorded as they were watching the pictures, allowing for an analysis of the distribution of their attention to the displayed stimuli. The findings showed that burnout and depression were associated with a similar tendency to overfocus on dysphoric stimuli and underfocus on positive stimuli. A study investigating memory functions found that burnout and depression predicted a similar pattern of alterations, consisting of an increased recall of negative items and a decreased recall of positive items (Bianchi, Laurent, et al., 2020). Studies of how ambiguous information is processed by people have documented that burnout and depression involve similar negative filters (Bianchi & da Silva Nogueira, 2019; Bianchi et al., 2018). People with burnout and depressive symptoms tend to favor negative interpretations of ambiguous content that could, with just as much plausibility, be interpreted positively. All in all, this body of research suggests that individuals with burnout symptoms process information and behave in ways that are characteristic of people with depressive symptoms.

Neurobiology of Burnout and Depression

Some investigators have suggested that neurobiological research would help to unambiguously distinguish burnout from depression. Cortisol, often referred to as the "stress hormone," became a focal concern in the quest for neurobiological markers of burnout (Bianchi et al., 2017; Rothe et al., 2020). A dichotomy started to emerge (e.g., Marchand et al., 2014). The dichotomy contrasted *hypo*cortisolism, that is, alterations involving deficits of cortisol, deemed to characterize burnout, with *hyper*cortisolism, that is, alterations involving excesses of cortisol, deemed to characterize depression. The dichotomy was meant to offer a basis for the burnout–depression distinction. The dichotomy, however, overlooked the fact that depression, depending on its subtypes and stages, can be accompanied by either hypo- or hypercortisolism (Bianchi et al., 2017; Gold & Chrousos, 2002; Lamers et al., 2013). For instance, depression with melancholic features has been associated with hypercortisolism, and depression with atypical features with hypocortisolism. We note that, despite its name, depression with atypical features is not rare. Historically, it was characterized as atypical because it contrasted with episodes of melancholic depression.[8]

Overall, research on the neurobiology of burnout and the identification of potential markers of the condition have been inconclusive (Jonsdottir & Sjörs Dahlman, 2019; Orosz et al., 2017; Rothe et al., 2020). Regarding cortisol, all sorts of profiles have eventually been observed, from hypocortisolism to normal cortisol metabolism and hypercortisolism. Recurrent limitations identified in systematic literature reviews (Jonsdottir & Sjörs Dahlman, 2019; Orosz et al., 2017;

---

8 As per the *DSM-5* (APA, 2013), depression with atypical features refers to a depressive episode accompanied by mood reactivity, that is, the mood of the affected person could at times brighten in response to a positive event or the anticipation of a positive event. Other symptoms can include increased appetite, hypersomnia, heavy feelings in the arms or legs, and heightened sensitivity to interpersonal rejection. Depression with melancholic features is marked by an almost total absence of pleasure in any activity. The reactivity observed in individuals with atypical depression is largely absent in individuals with melancholic depression. Other symptoms of depression with melancholic features can include profound despondency, dysphoric mood being particularly worse in the morning, waking up much earlier than unusual, anorexia, and excessive guilt.

Rothe et al., 2020) include (1) inconsistencies in the conceptualization and operationalization of burnout, (2) the neglect of potential confounders, and (3) an oversimplistic view of depressive conditions. It should be underlined that research on molecules such as cortisol is challenging given the complexity inherent in hormonal functioning. As an illustration, cortisol is not merely an effector of the stress response. Cortisol is involved in the regulation of the body's circadian rhythms—it usually peaks in the early morning to prepare the individual for action and gradually falls throughout the day, reaching its lowest levels at night. This aspect of cortisol's day-to-day activity has to be disentangled from the role of cortisol in the stress response as one usually understands it in stress research.

Anxiety and Depressive Symptoms

In Chapter 1, we noted that anxiety symptoms often co-occur with major depression. In that chapter, we also described an alternative to the categorical/diagnostic approach to depression. We underlined research that indicates that depressive and anxiety symptoms are important constituents of an internalizing dimension of psychopathology. In a study of U.S. schoolteachers (Schonfeld et al., 2019b), we built upon the idea that an anxio-depressive continuum of ill-being can be examined in relation to burnout.

We employed two standard measures of depressive symptoms, a ten-item version of the Center for Epidemiological Studies Depression scale (CESD-10)[9] and the PHQ-9, the 7-item Generalized Anxiety Disorder scale (GAD-7), and the MBI. We looked closely at the results bearing on the MBI-related syndromal hypothesis. As shown in Table 3.3, the syndromal hypothesis did not withstand the test. EE was more closely related to each of the two depressive symptom scales and the anxiety symptom scale than to DP and PA. Moreover, the correlations shown in the table barely changed when we recreated the depression scales by deleting items reflecting fatigue and sleep problems.

---

9 There is also the original 20-item version that we declined to use because the 10-item version we employed is very good from a psychometric standpoint and, with its fewer items, is less burdensome on respondents.

Table 3.3 The Pearson correlations are presented for the depressive and anxiety symptom scales and the MBI subscales.

Measures	CESD-10	CESD-9	PHQ-9	PHQ-7	GAD-7	EE	DP	PA	Job adversity
CESD-9	.97								
PHQ-9	.80	.77							
PHQ-7	.81	.79	.98						
GAD-7	.72	.70	.78	.75					
EE	.76	.74	.74	.71	.69				
DP	.56	.55	.54	.54	.50	.60			
PA	−.44	−.38	−.46	−.46	−.33	−.44	−.48		
Job adversity	.29	.30	.31	.32	.28	.36	.42	−.28	
Workplace support	−.39	−.40	−.40	−.40	−.38	−.42	−.34	.27	−.22

Note: CESD-10 = 10-item version of the left for Epidemiologic Studies Depression scale; CESD-9 = CESD with its only fatigue-related item deleted (see the text); PHQ-9 = Patient Health Questionnaire; PHQ-7 = Patient Health Questionnaire with the sleep-problems and fatigue items deleted (see the text); GAD-7 = 7-item Generalized Anxiety Disorder scale. EE = Emotional Exhaustion subscale of the Maslach Burnout Inventory (MBI). DP = Depersonalization subscale of the MBI. PA = Personal Accomplishment subscale of the MBI. All correlations are significant at $p < .001$. (Adapted from Schonfeld et al., 2019b).

We also built into the study a small nomological network component. The table shows that the depressive and anxiety symptom scales and EE (and DP and PA) were similarly related to job adversity and workplace support.

We extended our analysis by employing a statistical procedure called exploratory structural equation modeling (ESEM) bifactor analysis. Without getting overly technical, an ESEM bifactor analysis can identify a general or prime factor that could potentially account for the correlations among all symptom items. The analysis also involves extracting several secondary factors (bifactors) that explain variability specific to sets of symptom items, variability that is unrelated to the general factor (bifactors are constrained to be uncorrelated with the general factor). In this analysis, we dedicated one bifactor to each set of (sub)scale items. The items on each (sub)scale were allowed to "load" on a specific bifactor along with the general factor.

The ESEM bifactor analysis was consistent with the foregoing correlational findings. The PHQ-9, CESD-10, GAD-7, and EE items loaded substantially on the general factor, which here represents psychological distress along the anxio-depressive continuum. The items had weaker loadings on their respective secondary factors. By contrast, the DP and PA items had a less clear relation to the general factor.[10]

Bianchi et al. (2021) undertook an ESEM bifactor analysis involving 14 different samples of respondents from various countries. The authors found that burnout did not exhibit the unity expected of a distinct syndrome. Exhaustion and depression items primarily loaded on a common, general factor.

De Beer et al. (2024a) conducted an ESEM bifactor study using data collected in four countries. At first glance, these authors' findings might appear to conflict with the findings previously enumerated. The authors found "a strong underlying global factor representing participants' levels of psychological distress, as well as the presence of equally strong specific factors supporting the distinctive nature of burnout and

---

10 We use this footnote to provide additional details. The DP items had about equal loadings on their bifactor and the general factor; however, the items' loadings on the general factor were lower than the loadings of the PHQ-9, CESD, GAD-7, and EE items on the general factor. The PA items also tended to have lower loadings on the general factor; the items' loadings tended to be higher on PA's bifactor.

depression." Unfortunately, De Beer et al. used a symptom measure, the Four-Dimensional Symptom Questionnaire (Terluin et al., 2004), that overlooked no fewer than two-thirds of the symptoms used in diagnosing major depression. With most of the features of depression omitted, the study design likely made burnout look somewhat distinct from depression. Such a study did not compare burnout with depression. It compared burnout with three of the nine symptoms of depression.

The Occupational Depression Inventory

Although the foregoing evidence suggests that the items on burnout scales reflect depression dimensionally, burnout measures like the MBI's subscales assess only some (e.g., like fatigue), but not all, symptoms of depression. Burnout scales do not assess several key depressive symptoms. Humans respond to unresolvable stress, including unresolvable job stress, with well-known depressive symptoms that call for the attention of clinicians (Pryce et al., 2011; Willner et al., 2013). These include anhedonia, depressed mood, psychomotor alterations, and cognitive impairment (Bianchi et al., 2021). Another important symptom that emerges in response to unresolvable job stress is suicidality (Howard et al., 2022). Assessing suicidal ideation can help identify workers who urgently need care (Center for Suicide Prevention, 2020). We add that there is no identified iatrogenic risk associated with assessing suicidal ideation (DeCou & Schumann, 2018). Depressive symptom scales such as the PHQ-9 assess suicidal thoughts, underscoring that suicidal ideation is one of the nine diagnostic criteria for MDD (APA, 2013).

In view of the weaknesses identified in the burnout construct and its measures, we decided to develop a measure of work-related depression (Bianchi & Schonfeld, 2020; Schonfeld & Bianchi, 2022). The measure is called the Occupational Depression Inventory (ODI; see the Appendix for the English and French versions of the ODI). In our estimation, the ODI has the potential to replace burnout scales and become one of the tools to be used by occupational health specialists to identify distressed workers in need of treatment. Unlike traditional depressive symptom scales, which are cause-neutral, the ODI asks respondents if they ascribe the emergence of a symptom to their job (e.g., "My work was so stressful that I could not enjoy the things I usually like doing"). The ODI comprises nine symptom items keyed to the symptom criteria in the *DSM-5* for diagnosing MDD. The items cover symptom frequency over the preceding two weeks. The instrument comes with an algorithm that enables a clinician or researcher to use the pattern of responses to arrive at a provisional diagnosis of MDD.[11] The ODI also has one additional item that asks respondents, in view of whatever symptoms they have experienced, about turnover intentions.

Using three samples, a French schoolteacher sample, a New Zealand schoolteacher sample, and a U.S. sample comprising respondents having a variety of occupations, we (Bianchi & Schonfeld, 2020) established the psychometric and structural validity of the instrument in each sample. Regarding psychometric validity, we adduced evidence showing that the scale measures what it is purported to measure, work-related depression. With regard to structural validity, we showed the scale is unidimensional, that is, that it is measuring one construct and not mixing together more than one. In addition to our efforts in France, New Zealand, and the U.S., we worked with many collaborators in establishing the validity of the ODI in several countries and in the language of each country, including Spain (Bianchi, Manzano-García, et al., 2022), South Africa (Hill et al., 2021), Brazil (Bianchi, Calixto Cavalcante, et al., 2023), Italy (Bianchi, Fiorilli, et al., 2022), Sweden (Jansson-Fröjmark et al., 2023), Ukraine (Golonka et al., 2024), Poland (Golonka et al., 2024), Australia (Sowden et al., 2022; Bianchi, Verkuilen, et al., 2023), Switzerland (Bianchi, Verkuilen, et al., 2023), Germany (Bianchi et al., 2024), and Iran (Kalani et al., 2024). Other goals attained with the ODI have included the establishment of measurement invariance across countries, languages, sexes, and age groups (Bianchi et al., 2024). Measurement invariance refers to scale items having similar meanings and being used in the same manner across groups of interest. Table 3.4 provides a summary of key properties of the ODI and, for comparison purposes, the MBI-GS, the version of the MBI that can be used with the widest variety of occupations. As of the writing of this book, the ODI has been used in 85 countries.

---

11 The algorithm generates provisional diagnoses. As mentioned earlier, to make a more definitive diagnosis, a clinician needs to interview the individual.

Table 3.4 How the Occupational Depression Inventory (ODI) compares to the Maslach Burnout Inventory-General Survey (MBI-GS).

Features	ODI	MBI
Clear scoring guide	✓	✓
Multiple languages	✓	✓
Assessment of suicidal thoughts	✓	0
Foundation in theory and clinical practice	✓	0
Solid psychometric and structural properties	✓	0
Measurement invariance across groups	✓	0
Brevity	✓	0
Combines dimensional and diagnostic approaches	✓	0
Aids in prevalence estimation	✓	0

Note: In view of the need to conserve space, we recommend that readers consult Bianchi et al. (2024) regarding measurement invariance in the ODI and De Beer et al. (2024b) regarding limitations to the establishment of measurement invariance in the MBI-GS.

We (Schonfeld & Bianchi, 2022) evaluated the syndromal hypothesis in the context of studies of the relation of the ODI to (1) the MBI's subscales in a sample of French schoolteachers and (2) the Copenhagen Burnout Inventory (CBI; Kristensen et al., 2005) in a sample of New Zealand schoolteachers. Although there are three versions of the CBI, we used the version that assessed work-related burnout.[12] Like the MBI EE subscale, the focal concern of the CBI is work-related "physical and psychological fatigue and exhaustion" (Kristensen et al., 2005). As shown in Table 3.5, the ODI–EE correlation was greater than the correlations among the three MBI subscales, contradicting the syndromal hypothesis. In addition, the correlation of the ODI and the CBI was approximately equal to that of ODI–EE correlation. The pattern of correlations barely changed when we removed the fatigue and sleep-problems items from

---

12 As mentioned in Chapter 2, there are also versions that pertain to personal burnout and client-related burnout that were not relevant to the study by Schonfeld and Bianchi (2022).

Table 3.5 The correlations among the Occupational Depression Inventory (ODI) and the three subscales of the Maslach Burnout Inventory (MBI) in a sample of French schoolteachers and the ODI's correlation with Copenhagen Burnout Inventory (CBI) in a sample of New Zealand schoolteachers.

	France			New Zealand
Measures	EE	DP	PA	CBI
ODI	.80	.33	−.44	.80
EE		.44	−.55	
DP			−.49	
ODI-7	.78	.33	−.43	.76

Note: ODI = Occupational Burnout Inventory; ODI-7 is the Occupational Depression Inventory with the sleep-problems and fatigue items deleted (see the text); EE = Emotional Exhaustion subscale of the Maslach Burnout Inventory (MBI); DP = Depersonalization subscale of the MBI; PA = Personal Accomplishment subscale of the MBI; CBI = Copenhagen Burnout Inventory; ODI-7 = the score on the ODI with the fatigue and sleep problems items omitted. (Adapted from Schonfeld & Bianchi, 2022).

the ODI. The important point is that correlational findings in the two countries were consistent.

Schonfeld and Bianchi (2022) also conducted two ESEM bifactor analyses, one for the MBI and ODI data collected in France and the other for the CBI and ODI data collected in New Zealand. With the French data, we found that the ODI items and the EE items aligned, strongly loading on the general factor without discernable differences in their high loadings. The items on the bifactors (scale-specific factors) tended to be small. The DP and PA items tended to load more highly on their respective bifactors than on the general factor. In the New Zealand sample, the CBI and ODI items loaded highly on the general factor with much smaller loadings on their respective bifactors.

Sowden et al. (2022) employed a confirmatory factor analysis (CFA) in a study of Australian schoolteachers. The CFA was used to create factors that were grounded in six (sub)scales: the ODI; the Physical Fatigue, Cognitive Weariness, and Emotional Exhaustion subscales of the Shirom–Melamed Burnout Measure (SMBM); and the Exhaustion and Disengagement subscales of the Oldenburg Burnout Inventory

(OLBI). Sowden et al. found that the Occupational Depression factor was highly correlated with the five other factors rooted in the subscales of the SMBM and OLBI. The Occupational Depression factor correlated more highly with the SMBM Physical Fatigue, Cognitive Weariness, and Emotional Exhaustion factors (mean $r = .67$) than the SMBM factors correlated with each other (mean $r = .57$). The Occupational Depression factor correlated about as highly with the OLBI Exhaustion and Disengagement factors (mean $r = .73$) as the two OLBI factors correlated with each other ($r = .72$). Taken together, these findings suggest that the SMBM and the OLBI subscales are mainly but imperfectly measuring depressive symptomatology, contradicting the syndromal hypothesis.

In a study of Brazilian civil servants, Bianchi, Calixto Cavalcante, et al. (2023) found that the 12-item version of the Burnout Assessment Tool (BAT-12; Schaufeli et al., 2020; Sinval et al., 2022) was highly correlated with the ODI ($r = .82$), suggesting that this burnout scale was measuring depression. The BAT-12 comprises four 3-item subscales (Exhaustion, Mental Distance, Cognitive Impairment, and Emotional Impairment). The investigators found that the subscales were more highly correlated with the ODI (mean $r = .68$) than with each other (mean $r = .57$), a finding consistent with a CFA applied to the data and contradicting the syndromal hypothesis.

Other Studies That Bear on Burnout–Depression Overlap

Research on doctors and dentists also ties burnout closely to depression. In a study of Austrian physicians, Wurm et al. (2016) found that the Emotional Exhaustion subscale of the Hamburg Burnout Inventory (HBI) correlated more highly with symptoms of depression (e.g., sadness, lack of interest) than with other components of the HBI (Personal Accomplishment, Detachment). Wurm et al. found that as the frequency of burnout symptoms increased, the risk of meeting criteria for major depression increased in parallel. Compared to physicians without burnout symptoms, physicians with severe burnout symptoms were at 93 times the risk of meeting criteria for a diagnosis of major depression.

In a longitudinal study of symptom clusters and their trajectories in Finnish dentists, Ahola et al. (2014) found that at the Time-1 baseline MBI and depressive symptoms tended to cluster in low-, medium-, and high-symptom groups. There were two follow-ups, with Time 2 three years later and Time 3 seven years after baseline. The investigators found that either the members of the three symptom groups remained about the same over time, or, if symptoms became more or less frequent, burnout and depressive symptoms changed in the same direction.

Ahola et al.'s (2014) findings were successfully replicated in a two-wave study of French schoolteachers (Bianchi et al., 2015a, b). Bianchi et al. (2015a) observed that burnout and depressive symptoms clustered both at the Time-1 baseline and 21 months later at follow-up. Changes in burnout and depressive symptoms from Time 1 to Time 2 overlapped: Teachers with increasing burnout symptoms experienced increases in depressive symptoms and teachers with decreasing burnout symptoms experienced decreases in depressive symptoms. Moreover, the researchers also found that burnout and depression were highly correlated at both Time 1 ($r = .64$) and Time 2 ($r = .68$). Relying on classical regression frameworks, Bianchi et al. (2015b) found that baseline burnout symptoms no longer predicted depressive symptoms at follow-up when baseline depressive symptoms were statistically controlled. These results illustrate the overlap of burnout with depression in yet another manner.

Rössler et al. (2015) examined the relation between scores on the MBI subscales and the subscales of the 90-item measure of psychopathology, known as the SCL-90R, in a sample of workers living in the canton of Zurich. The researchers found that EE correlated with depressive symptoms .50. The correlation, however, should be interpreted with caution because the sample was greatly unbalanced, with two-thirds of the participant pool having been selected because they had high psychopathology scores, reducing variability in the sample, which may have the effect of lowering correlation coefficients. In addition, there was no information on how the EE–depression correlation compared to the correlations among the MBI's subscales. Interestingly, not just the depression scale but every other psychopathology scale (e.g., anxiety, psychoticism) correlated significantly with EE. In addition, a lifetime history of mood disorder (e.g., depression) was related to EE.

Meta-analyses

The foregoing studies provide a flavor for the research on burnout–depression overlap. Meta-analyses, however, provide a more commanding view of the burnout–depression landscape. To our knowledge, there have been five meta-analyses bearing on the magnitude of the correlation between burnout scales and depressive symptom scales (Bianchi et al., 2021; Koutsimani et al., 2019; Meier & Kim, 2022; Schonfeld et al., 2019a; Swingler et al., 2023). We examine them in chronological order.

Schonfeld et al. (2019a) conducted a meta-analysis pertaining to burnout and depression that covered 13 studies and 15 separate samples of diverse workers. The meta-analysis was limited to studies that used the MBI and were published during the ten years preceding publication (as per the suggestion of a reviewer). The results bearing on the syndromal hypothesis are shown in Table 3.6. Contrary to what the syndromal hypothesis would predict, the EE–depression correlation was higher than the correlations among the MBI subscales, EE, DP, and PA (see Table 3.6). The EE-depression correlation averaged .60. When we adjusted for measurement error, it was estimated to be .70.

The meta-analysis Koutsimani et al. (2019) conducted involved 67 studies and 69 separate samples. Although not limited to the MBI, the MBI was the most used burnout measure in the meta-analysis. Key correlations extracted from the study are in Table 3.7. The mean burnout–depression and EE–depression correlations were slightly

Table 3.6 Correlations found in the 15-sample meta-analysis.

Measures	No. of samples	r
Emotional Exhaustion–Depression	15	.60
Emotional Exhaustion–Depersonalization	12	.49
Depersonalization–Personal Accomplishment	8	−.29
Emotional Exhaustion–Personal Accomplishment	8	−.30
Depersonalization–Depression	13	.40
Personal Accomplishment–Depression	11	−.33

Adapted from Schonfeld et al. (2019a).

Table 3.7 Key findings from the meta-analysis conducted.

Measures	r
Depression–MBI	.52
Depression–EE	.51
Depression–average of DP and PA	.41
Depression–non-MBI measures	.75
PHQ-9–Burnout	.63

Note: MBI = Maslach Burnout Inventory (MBI); EE = Emotional Exhaustion subscale of the MBI; DP = Depersonalization subscale of the MBI; PA = Personal Accomplishment subscale of the MBI; PHQ-9 is the nine-item Patient Health Questionnaire measure of depressive symptoms. Adapted from Koutsimani et al. (2019).

above .50, higher than the mean correlation of depression with DP and PA (only the average of the two correlations was reported). In studies that reported total burnout scores by using non-MBI scales, burnout correlated .75 with depressive symptoms. When depressive symptoms were assessed with the PHQ-9, which in many ways is the best validated depression symptom scale available (Bianchi, Verkuilen, et al., 2022), the mean burnout–depression correlation was. .63. The results of the meta-analysis do not bear on the syndromal hypothesis because the mean EE–depression correlation was not compared to the average correlations among the MBI subscales, EE, DP, and PA, or their surrogates found in non-MBI studies. Another limitation of the meta-analysis is that the authors did not calculate correlations that were corrected for measurement error (the disattenuated correlations).

A consortium of investigators pooled 14 different samples from six countries to conduct a meta-analysis relevant to testing the syndromal hypothesis (Bianchi et al., 2021). Table 3.8 summarizes the results of the meta-analysis. The disattenuated correlation between Exhaustion and Depression was .80. The table shows that, contrary to the syndromal hypothesis, Exhaustion is more closely related to depressive symptoms than to Detachment (a stand-in for Depersonalization and Cynicism) or Personal Accomplishment.

Table 3.8 The meta-analytically pooled disattenuated correlations from the 14-sample meta-analysis.

Measures	Disattenuated correlations
Depression–Exhaustion	.80
Depression–Detachment	.53
Depression–Efficacy	–.47
Exhaustion–Detachment	.64
Exhaustion–Efficacy	–.43
Detachment–Efficacy	–.45

Note: The detachment construct embraces both depersonalization and cynicism. It reflects the mental distancing thought to characterize someone with burnout. Efficacy reflects personal accomplishment and efficacy at work. Adapted from Bianchi et al. (2021).

Meier and Kim (2022) conducted a meta-analysis of 69 studies and 74 samples. The investigators found that the mean correlation between burnout and depression was .49, close to the mean correlation of .52 that Koutsimani et al. (2019) obtained. Meier and Kim also found that the MBI EE–depression correlation averaged .55; however, they did not test the syndromal hypothesis. There were no comparisons between the EE–depression correlation, on one hand, to the correlations among the MBI subscales, on the other. And disattenuated correlations were not computed.

Additionally, Meier and Kim (2022) observed that "[t]ypically around .50, this correlation has been interpreted as both supporting and negating the distinctiveness of burnout when compared to depression" (p. 201). They noted that in the research literature on psychological measures, "evidence of convergent validity" is found with correlations ranging from .50 to .60.

A factor that limits the size of burnout–depression correlations, according to Meier and Kim (2022), is that "contemporary burnout measures include item content related to work, while depression measures do not" (p. 202). They noted that this limitation could be mitigated by researchers adopting Bianchi and Schonfeld's (2020) ODI. Indeed, three studies mentioned earlier in this chapter, Schonfeld and

Bianchi (2022), Bianchi, Calixto Cavalcante et al. (2023), and Sowden et al. (2022), found that the ODI demonstrated high correlations with the MBI's EE subscale, the CBI, the BAT, and the SMBM. By the same token, we observe that the periods covered by burnout and depression scales also mitigate against higher correlations. The MBI covers the frequency of burnout symptoms over the year while depressive symptom scales such as the PHQ-9 and ODI cover the previous two weeks and the CESD covers one week.

The fifth and most recent meta-analysis on burnout–depression correlations was conducted by Swingler et al. (2023). Unlike the other two large meta-analyses (Koutsimani et al., 2019 and Meier & Kim, 2022), Swingler et al. assessed the reliability of the coding scheme used to identify studies that met inclusion criteria. Two raters independently judged 140 studies (half relevant to the meta-analysis and half not). The coefficient of agreement, kappa, was .85, and regarded as acceptable. With 96 samples, the investigators addressed the syndromal hypothesis. When non-MBI (sub)scales were used, they were matched to the MBI subscales. For example, like the MBI's EE subscale, the CBI and the OLBI's Exhaustion subscale were treated as reflecting Exhaustion. Like the MBI's DP subscale, the OLBI's Disengagement subscale was treated as reflecting Detachment.

As shown in Table 3.9, the mean Exhaustion–Depression correlation was stronger than the mean correlations among the Exhaustion, Detachment, and Efficacy measures. The application of Duval and Tweedie's (2000) trim-and-fill procedure, which adjusts for bias owing to missing studies, that is, the "file drawer problem" (Rosenthal, 1979; also see Chapter 5), produced adjusted mean correlations; most were adjusted upward and one, downward (see Table 3.9). The table also includes the disattenuated correlations, which also underline the closeness of Exhaustion to Depression. The patterning of the adjusted correlations, however, was similar to that of the raw correlations. Thus, the syndromal hypothesis did not hold.

For a statistical reason mentioned in the section of Chapter 2 on correlation and reliability coefficients, each disattenuated correlation involving Detachment is likely biased upward (compared to the correlations not involving Detachment) because the measures of Detachment were considerably less reliable (had lower reliability coefficients) than

Table 3.9 The results of the 96-sample meta-analysis.

Dimensions correlated	No. of studies	Correlations	Trim-and-fill adjusted correlations	Disattentuated correlations
Depression–Exhaustion	96	.60	.66	.68
Depression–Detachment	84	.43	.44	.53
Depression–Efficacy	62	.32	.37	.38
Exhaustion–Detachment	72	.56	.54	.68
Exhaustion–Efficacy	51	.28	.35	.33
Detachment–Efficacy	50	.36	.38	.46

Note: Detachment includes both "depersonalization" and "cynicism." Efficacy reflects "personal accomplishment" and "professional efficacy." To be consistent with the negative direction of higher scores on the scales assessing Exhaustion, Detachment, and Depression, Efficacy was reversed scored such that higher scores reflect a worse sense of personal accomplishment and professional efficacy. Adapted from Swingler et al. (2023).

the other measures. This phenomenon can be observed in the discrepancy between, on one hand, the disattenuated Exhaustion–Detachment correlation and, on the other, the trim-and-fill corrected correlation. There is a parallel discrepancy between the disattenuated Depression–Detachment correlation and the trim-and-fill corrected correlation. We advise readers to use caution when looking at disattenuated correlations involving Detachment.

Conclusions

The preponderance of evidence indicates that, if anything, burnout reflects a depressive phenomenon. The evidence we outlined begins with Herbert Freudenberger. In 1974, he observed the similarity between burnout and depression when he first attempted to describe burnout. It then took several years for research on burnout–depression to catch up. In 1984, Scott T. Meier, in a study of university faculty, found that three burnout measures and depressive symptom scales were about equally correlated with each other, suggesting burnout–depression overlap. We noted that the foundational measurement ideas of discriminant validity (Campbell & Fiske, 1959) dovetailed with the syndromal hypothesis, namely, the burnout scales assessing exhaustion, depersonalization (or detachment or cynicism), and reduced personal accomplishment (or inefficacy) should be more closely correlated with each other than with measures of different constructs (Bianchi et al., 2021; Schonfeld & Bianchi, 2021a, b). Of course, the key different construct of interest here has been depression.

The research literature tells us that there are two complementary ways of conceptualizing depression, as a phenomenon that is either present or absent or as a dimensional phenomenon that varies on a continuum. We explored the relation of burnout to both conceptualizations of depression (Bianchi et al., 2013, 2014; Schonfeld & Bianchi, 2016), finding that burnout is strongly related to depression in either conceptualization. We found high correlations of burnout symptoms with depressive symptoms measured dimensionally (Bianchi et al., 2013, 2014; Schonfeld & Bianchi, 2016) although other investigators have found lower—but still large—correlations (e.g., Meier & Kim, 2022). The research literature also indicated that individuals who experience burnout symptoms on a (near-)daily basis are likely to meet the criteria for a current diagnosis of depression or have a history of mood disorder (Bianchi et al., 2013, 2014; Rössler et al., 2015; Schonfeld & Bianchi, 2016; Wurm et al., 2016).

We also investigated the nomological networks of burnout and depression. We found close parallels in the relationships of burnout and depression to other key variables. Burnout and depressive symptoms are related to essentially the same factors, inside and outside of the workplace, for example, work-related support from coworkers and stressful life events occurring outside of work. Burnout and depression are associated with similar cognitive and behavioral alterations. Such close parallels are not expected if dealing with distinct conditions. Once thought to settle the idea of a distinction between burnout and depression, research on cortisol has not provided conclusive evidence.

Evidence from well-controlled longitudinal studies described in Chapter 1 demonstrates that adverse working conditions can increase depression risk. Adverse working conditions can also lead to increased burnout symptoms. Sen (2022) in the pages of the *New England Journal of Medicine* observed: "the argument that depression and burnout are caused by fundamentally different precipitants is unsupported by the evidence to date" (p. 1630). The parallel in precipitants, along with the invalidity of the syndromal hypothesis, suggests that burnout reflects a depressive condition.

ESEM bifactor analyses are also consistent with the idea that the exhaustion component of burnout aligns with depressive symptoms (Bianchi et al., 2021; Schonfeld et al., 2019a; Verkuilen et al., 2021). These studies have found that EE symptom items load just as strongly on the general factor as depressive symptom items and have weaker loadings on their respective bifactors. By contrast, DP and PA items tend to have stronger loadings on their bifactors and, compared to EE items, weaker loadings on the general factor. When we conducted CFAs (Bianchi, Verkuilen, & Schonfeld, 2020; Schonfeld et al., 2019a) in eight different samples, we obtained very high Exhaustion–Depression factor correlations. These studies found additional evidence that contradicts the syndromal hypothesis.

We also described five meta-analyses. Of particular interest are the exhaustion–depression correlations because the evidence points to exhaustion-related burnout (sub)scales being the burnout scales that most reflect depression. We use the term "exhaustion" because we grouped together MBI EE subscales with non-MBI (sub)scales that also reflected exhaustion. The two smaller meta-analyses obtained exhaustion–depression correlations shorn of measurement error of .70 (Schonfeld et al., 2019a) and .80 (Bianchi et al., 2021). In two larger meta-analyses, one mean EE–depression correlation was .51 (Koutsimani et al., 2019), and the other was .55 (Meier & Kim, 2022), which, when disattenuated, we estimate to range from .60 to .65. In the third large meta-analysis (Swingler et al., 2023), the exhaustion–depression correlation was .60; adjusted it was .66 or .68 depending upon which type of adjustment was used.

In three of the meta-analyses (Bianchi et al., 2021; Schonfeld et al., 2019a; Swingler et al., 2023), the adjusted exhaustion–depression correlations were higher than .60; in two of the meta-analysis (Koutsimani et al., 2019; Meier & Kim, 2022), the correlations were not adjusted for measurement error or by way of the trim-and-fill procedure. Two of the meta-analyses (Koutsimani et al., 2019; Meier & Kim, 2022) did not test the syndromal hypothesis. Three (Bianchi et al., 2021; Schonfeld et al., 2019a; Swingler et al., 2023), however, did. In each of the three cases, the findings contradicted the syndromal hypothesis, suggesting that the exhaustion dimension of burnout is closer to depression than to other burnout subscales.

Meier and Kim (2022) suggested that one way to improve our understanding of the relationship between burnout and depression may be to use a depression scale that, like burnout scales, is concerned with symptoms that are work-related. They referred to the ODI (Bianchi & Schonfeld, 2020; Schonfeld & Bianchi, 2022). We used the ODI to test the syndromal hypothesis in several countries, including France and New Zealand (Schonfeld & Bianchi, 2022), Australia (Sowden et al., 2022), and Brazil (Bianchi, Calixto Cavalcante, et al., 2023). The ODI studies show that the core exhaustion symptom component of burnout was more closely related to depression than to the other putative components of burnout.

We have also learned of two kinds of speculation (Schonfeld, 2021b). One is that burnout symptoms mediate the relation of job stressors to depressive symptoms. The other is that depressive symptoms mediate the relation of job stressors to burnout. Thus, in one way of thinking, job stressors precipitate an increase in burnout symptoms, which, in turn, give rise to depressive symptoms. In another way of thinking, job stressors precipitate an increase in depressive symptoms, which in turn give rise to burnout symptoms. However, such speculation is specious because the discriminant validity of burnout vis-à-vis depression has not been established.

The importance of understanding that burnout is a depressive phenomenon cannot be overstated. If a worker is identified as "burned out," a well-intentioned colleague or friend may recommend a vacation. A problem with the recommendation of a vacation for a burned-out individual is that a vacation's beneficial impact will likely have faded a few weeks after the individual has returned to work (de Bloom et al., 2009; Kühnel & Sonnentag, 2011; Reizer & Mey-Raz, 2019; Westman & Etzion, 2001).

An important concern is that the burnout label can mask depression. There is a good chance that the dysphoria affecting the worker identified as burned out will endure. Moreover, depression is comorbid with many physical diseases, including cardiovascular disease and neurological disorders, and is associated with reduced life expectancy (Berk et al., 2023). Stressful job conditions are associated with higher levels of suicidal ideation (Niedhammer et al., 2024). Depression increases the risk of attempted (Dong et al., 2019) and completed suicide (Berman, 2009). Thus, letting depression go untreated because it is masked by the facile label of burnout can have terrible ramifications. It is important to get the affected worker into treatment with a skilled clinician who understands depression. Interventions to help people with depression include psychotherapy and pharmacotherapy. One key objective of the therapeutic process is to identify the factors that lead to the development of depression. One of those factors is adverse job conditions. We cover two types of psychotherapy in Chapter 5. We also review organizational interventions that can be implemented to reduce work-related psychological distress (see Chapter 5).

References

Ahola, K., Hakanen, J., Perhoniemi, R., & Mutanen, P. (2014). Relationship between burnout and depressive symptoms: A study using the person-centred approach. *Burnout Research*, *1*(1), 29–37. https://doi.org/10.1016/j.burn.2014.03.003

Ahola, K., Honkonen, T., Isometsä, E., Kalimo, R., Nykyri, E., Aromaa, A., & Lönnqvist, J. (2005). The relationship between job-related burnout and depressive disorders—Results from the Finnish Health 2000 Study. *Journal of Affective Disorders*, *88*, 55–62. https://doi.org/10.1016/j.jad.2005.06.004

American Psychiatric Association. (2013). *Diagnostic and statistical manual of mental disorders*, (5th ed.). Author. https://www.psychiatry.org/psychiatrists/practice/dsm

Bakker, A. B., Schaufeli, W. B., Demerouti, E., Janssen, P. P. M., Van Der Hulst, R., & Brouwer, J. (2000). Using equity theory to examine the difference between burnout and depression. *Anxiety, Stress, & Coping*, *13*(3), 247–268. https://doi.org/10.1080/10615800008549265

Beck, A. T., Ward, C. H., Mendelson, M., Mock, J., & Erbaugh, J. (1961). An inventory for measuring depression. *Archives of General Psychiatry*, *4*, 561–571. https://doi-org.ezproxy.gc.cuny.edu/10.1001/archpsyc.1961.01710120031004

Berk, M., Köhler-Forsberg, O., Turner, M., Penninx, B. W. J. H., Wrobel, A., Firth, J., Loughman, A., Reavley, N. J., McGrath, J. J., Momen, N. C., Plana-Ripoll, O., O'Neil, A., Siskind, D., Williams, L. J., Carvalho, A. F., Schmaal, L., Walker, A. J., Dean, O., Walder, K., ... Marx, W. (2023). Comorbidity between major depressive disorder and physical diseases: A comprehensive review of epidemiology, mechanisms and management. *World Psychiatry*, *22*(3), 366–387. https://doi.org/10.1002/wps.21110

Berman, A. L. (2009). Depression and suicide. In I. H. Gotlib and C. L. Hammen (Eds.), *Handbook of depression* (2nd ed.), (pp. 508–530). Guilford.

Bianchi, R., & da Silva Nogueira, D. (2019). Burnout is associated with a depressive interpretation style. *Stress and Health*, *35*(5), 642–649. https://doi.org/10.1002/smi.2897

Bianchi, R., & Laurent, E. (2015). Emotional information processing in depression and burnout: An eye-tracking study. *European Archives of Psychiatry and Clinical Neuroscience*, *265*(1), 27–34. https://doi.org/10.1007/s00406-014-0549-x

Bianchi, R., & Schonfeld, I. S. (2016). Burnout is associated with a depressive cognitive style. *Personality and Individual Differences*, *100*, 1–5. https://doi.org/10.1016/j.paid.2016.01.008

Bianchi, R., & Schonfeld, I. S. (2020). The Occupational Depression Inventory: A new tool for clinicians and epidemiologists. *Journal of Psychosomatic Research*, *138*, 110249. https://doi.org/10.1016/j.jpsychores.2020.110249

Bianchi, R., & Schonfeld, I. S. (2023). Examining the evidence base for burnout. *Bulletin of the World Health Organization*, *101*, 743–745. http://dx.doi.org/10.2471/BLT.23.289996

Bianchi, R., & Schonfeld, I. S. (2024). Beliefs about burnout. *Work & Stress*. http://dx.doi.org/10.1080/02678373.2024.2364590

Bianchi, R., Boffy, C., Hingray, C., Truchot, D., & Laurent, E. (2013). Comparative symptomatology of burnout and depression. *Journal of Health Psychology*, *18*(6), 782–787. https://doi.org/10.1177/1359105313481079

Bianchi, R., Calixto Cavalcante, D., Queirós, C., Menezes Santos, B. D., & Schonfeld, I. S. (2023). Validation of the Occupational Depression Inventory in Brazil: A study of 1,612 civil servants. *Journal of Psychosomatic Research*, *167*, 111194. https://doi.org/10.1016/j.jpsychores.2023.111194

Bianchi, R., Fiorilli, C., Angelini, G., Dozio, N., Palazzi, C., Palazzi, G., Vitiello, B., & Schonfeld, I. S. (2022). Occupational depression in Italy: Associations with health, economic, and work-life characteristics. *Frontiers in Psychiatry, 13*, 061293. https://doi.org/10.3389/fpsyt.2022.1061293

Bianchi, R., Laurent, E., Schonfeld, I. S., Bietti, L. M., & Mayor, E. (2020). Memory bias toward emotional information in burnout and depression. *Journal of Health Psychology, 25*(10-11), 1567-1575. https://doi.org/10.1177/1359105318765621

Bianchi, R., Laurent, E., Schonfeld, I. S., Verkuilen, J., & Berna, C. (2018). Interpretation bias toward ambiguous information in burnout and depression. *Personality and Individual Differences, 135*, 216-221. https://doi.org/10.1016/j.paid.2018.07.028

Bianchi, R., Manzano-García, G., Montañés Muro, M. P., Schonfeld, E. A., & Schonfeld, I. S. (2022). Occupational depression in a Spanish-speaking sample: Associations with cognitive performance and work-life characteristics. *Journal of Work and Organizational Psychology, 38*(1), 59-74. https://doi.org/10.5093/jwop2022a5

Bianchi, R., Schonfeld, I. S., & Laurent, E. (2014). Is burnout a depressive disorder? A reexamination with special focus on atypical depression. *International Journal of Stress Management, 21*, 307-324. https://doi.org/10.1037/a0037906

Bianchi, R., Schonfeld, I. S., & Laurent, E. (2015a). Is burnout separable from depression in cluster analysis? A longitudinal study. *Social Psychiatry and Psychiatric Epidemiology, 50*(6), 1005-1011. https://doi.org/10.1007/s00127-014-0996-8

Bianchi, R., Schonfeld, I. S., & Laurent, E. (2015b). Burnout does not help predict depression in French schoolteachers. *Scandinavian Journal of Work, Environment & Health, 41*(6), 565-568. http://dx.doi.org/10.5271/sjweh.3522

Bianchi, R., Schonfeld, I. S., & Laurent, E. (2017). Biological research on burnout-depression overlap: Long-standing limitations and on-going reflections. *Neuroscience & Biobehavioral Reviews, 83*, 238-239. https://doi.org/10.1016/j.neubiorev.2017.10.019

Bianchi, R., Schonfeld, I. S., & Verkuilen, J. (2020). A five-sample confirmatory factor analytic study of burnout-depression overlap. *Journal of Clinical Psychology, 76*, 801-821. http://dx.doi.org/10.1002/jclp.22927

Bianchi, R., Schonfeld, I. S., Sowden, J. F., Cavalcante, D. C., Queirós, C., Hebel, V. M., Volmer, J., Fiorilli, C., Angelini, G., Golonka, K., Manzano-García, G., Montañés-Muro, P., Jansson-Fröjmark, M., & De Beer, L. T. (2024). Measurement invariance of the Occupational Depression Inventory: A study of 12,589 participants across 14 countries. *Work & Stress*. Advance online publication. https://doi.org/10.1080/02678373.2024.2364594

Bianchi, R., Verkuilen, J., Schonfeld, I. S., Hakanen, J. J., Jansson-Fröjmark, M., Manzano-García, G., Laurent, E., & Meier, L. L. (2021). Is burnout a depressive condition? A 14-sample meta-analytic and bifactor analytic study. *Clinical Psychological Science, 9*(4), 579–597. https://doi.org/10.1177/2167702620979597

Bianchi, R., Verkuilen, J., Sowden, J., & Schonfeld, I. S. (2023). Toward a new approach to job-related distress: A three-sample study of the Occupational Depression Inventory. *Stress & Health, 39*(1), 137–153. https://doi.org/10.1002/smi.3177

Bianchi, R., Verkuilen, J., Toker, S., Schonfeld, I. S., Gerber, M., Brähler, E., & Kroenke, K. (2022). Is the PHQ-9 a unidimensional measure of depression? A 58,272-participant study. *Psychological Assessment, 34*(6), 595–603. https://doi.org/10.1037/pas0001124

Campbell, D. T., & Fiske, D. W. (1959). Convergent and discriminant validation by the multitrait-multimethod matrix. *Psychological Bulletin, 56*(2), 81–105. https://doi.org/10.1037/h0046016

Center for Suicide Prevention. (2020). The workplace and suicide prevention. https://www.suicideinfo.ca/resource/workplace-suicide-prevention/

Cronbach, L. J., & Meehl, P. E. (1955). Construct validity in psychological tests. *Psychological Bulletin, 52*(4), 281–302. https://doi.org/10.1037/h0040957

De Beer, L. T., Hakanen, J. J., Schaufeli, W. B., De Witte, H., Glaser, J., Kaltiainen, J., Seubert, C., & Morin, A. J. S. (2024a). The burnout-depression conundrum: Investigating construct-relevant multidimensionality across four countries and four patient samples. *Psychology & Health*, 1–28. Advance online publication. https://doi.org/10.1080/08870446.2024.2321358

De Beer, L. T., van der Vaart, L., Escaffi-Schwarz, M., De Witte, H., & Schaufeli, W. B. (2024b). Maslach Burnout Inventory—General Survey: A systematic review and meta-analysis of measurement properties.

European Journal of Psychological Assessment. *40*(5), 360–375. Advance online publication. https://doi.org/10.1027/1015-5759/a000797

de Bloom, J., Kompier, M., Geurts, S., de Weerth, C., Taris, T., & Sonnentag, S. (2009). Do we recover from vacation? Meta-analysis of vacation effects on health and well-being. *Journal of Occupational Health*, *51*(1), 13–25. http://dx.doi.org/10.1539/joh.K8004

DeCou, C. R., & Schumann, M. E. (2018). On the iatrogenic risk of assessing suicidality: A meta-analysis. *Suicide and Life-Threatening Behavior*, *48*(5), 531–543. https://doi.org/10.1111/sltb.12368

Dong, M., Zeng, L.-N., Lu, L., Li, X.-H., Ungvari, G. S., Ng, C. H., Chow, I. H. I., Zhang, L., Zhou, Y., & Xiang, Y.-T. (2019). Prevalence of suicide attempt in individuals with major depressive disorder: A meta-analysis of observational surveys. *Psychological Medicine*, *49*(10), 1691–1704. https://doi.org/10.1017/S0033291718002301

Duval, S., & Tweedie, R. (2000). Trim and fill: A simple funnel-plot-based method of testing and adjusting for publication bias in meta-analysis. *Biometrics*, *56*(2), 455–463. https://doi.org/10.1111/j.0006-341X.2000.00455.x

Freudenberger, H. J. (1974). Staff burnout. *Journal of Social Issues*, *30*(1), 159–165. https://doi.org/10.1111/j.1540-4560.1974.tb00706.x

Gold, P. W., & Chrousos, G. P. (2002). Organization of the stress system and its dysregulation in melancholic and atypical depression: High vs low CRH/NE states. *Molecular Psychiatry*, *7*(3), 254–275. https://doi.org/10.1038/sj.mp.4001032

Golonka, K., Malysheva, K. O., Fortuna, D., Gulla, B., Lytvyn, S., De Beer, L. T., Schonfeld, I. S., & Bianchi, R. (2024). A validation study of the Occupational Depression Inventory in Poland and Ukraine. *Scientific Reports*, *14*(1), 4403. https://doi.org/10.1038/s41598-024-54995-w

Guthier, C., Dormann, C., & Voelkle, M. C. (2020). Reciprocal effects between job stressors and burnout: A continuous time meta-analysis of longitudinal studies. *Psychological Bulletin*, *146*(12), 1146–1173. https://doi.org/10.1037/bul0000304

Hill, C., De Beer, L. T., & Bianchi, R. (2021). Validation and measurement invariance of the Occupational Depression Inventory in South Africa. *PLoS ONE*, *16*(12), e0261271. https://doi.org/10.1371/journal.pone.0261271

Howard, M. C., Follmer, K. B., Smith, M. B., Tucker, R. P., & Van Zandt, E. C. (2022). Work and suicide: An interdisciplinary systematic literature review.

Journal of Organizational Behavior, 43(2), 260–285. https://doi.org/10.1002/job.2519

Jansson-Fröjmark, M., Badinlou, F., Lundgren, T., Schonfeld, I.S., & Bianchi, R. (2023). Validation of the occupational depression inventory in Sweden. *BMC Public Health, 23*(1). https://doi.org/10.1186/s12889-023-16417-w

Jonsdottir, I. H., & Sjörs Dahlman, A. (2019). Mechanisms in endocrinology. Endocrine and immunological aspects of burnout: A narrative review. *European Journal of Endocrinology, 180*(3), R147–R158. https://doi.org/10.1530/eje-18-0741

Kalani, S., Khanlari, P., & Bianchi, R. (2024). A Persian Validation of the Occupational Depression Inventory. *European Journal of Psychological Assessment*. https://doi.org/10.1027/1015-5759/a000830

Koutsimani, P., Montgomery, A., & Georganta, K. (2019). The relationship between burnout, depression, and anxiety: A systematic review and meta-analysis. *Frontiers in Psychology, 10*, Article 284. https://doi.org/10.3389/fpsyg.2019.00284

Kristensen, T. S., Borritz, M., Villadsen, E., & Christensen, K. B. (2005). The Copenhagen Burnout Inventory: A new tool for the assessment of burnout. *Work and Stress, 19*, 192–207. https://doi.org/10.1080/02678370500297720

Kroenke, K., Spitzer, R. L., & Williams, J. B. W. (2001). The PHQ-9: Validity of a brief depression severity measure. *Journal of General Internal Medicine, 16*(9), 606–613. https://doi.org/10.1046/j.1525-1497.2001.016009606.x

Kühnel, J., & Sonnentag, S. (2011). How long do you benefit from vacation? A closer look at the fade-out of vacation effects. *Journal of Organizational Behavior, 32*(1), 125–143. https://doi.org/10.1002/job.699

Lamers, F., Vogelzangs, N., Merikangas, K. R., de Jonge, P., Beekman, A. T. F., & Penninx, B. W. J. H. (2013). Evidence for a differential role of HPA-axis function, inflammation and metabolic syndrome in melancholic versus atypical depression. *Molecular Psychiatry, 18*(6), 692–699. https://doi.org/10.1038/mp.2012.144

Leiter, M. P., & Durup, J. (1994). The discriminant validity of burnout and depression: A confirmatory factor analytic study. *Anxiety, Stress, and Coping, 7*, 357–373. http://dx.doi.org/10.1080/10615809408249357

Marchand, A., Durand, P., Juster, R. P., & Lupien, S. J. (2014). Workers' psychological distress, depression, and burnout symptoms: Associations with diurnal cortisol profiles. *Scandinavian Journal of Work, Environment & Health, 40*(3), 305–314. https://doi.org/10.5271/sjweh.3417

Maslach, C. (1976). Burned-out. *Human Behavior: The Newsmagazine of the Social Sciences, 5*(9), 16–22.

Maslach, C., & Leiter, M. P. (2016). Understanding the burnout experience: Recent research and its implications for psychiatry. *World Psychiatry, 15*, 103–111. https://doi.org/10.1002/wps.20311

Maslach, C., Jackson, S. E., & Leiter, M. P. (1996). *Maslach Burnout Inventory Manual* (3rd ed.). Consulting Psychologists Press.

Maslach, C., Schaufeli, W. B., & Leiter, M. P. (2001). Job burnout. *Annual Review of Psychology, 52*(1), 397–422. https://doi.org/10.1146/annurev.psych.52.1.397

Meier, S. T. (1984). The construct validity of burnout. *Journal of Occupational Psychology, 53*(3), 211–219. https://doi.org/10.1111/j.2044-8325.1984.tb00163.x

Meier, S. T., & Kim, S. (2022). Meta-regression analyses of relationships between burnout and depression with sampling and measurement methodological moderators. *Journal of Occupational Health Psychology, 27*(2), 195–206. https://doi.org/10.1037/ocp0000273

Melnick, E. R., Powsner, S. M., & Shanafelt, T. D. (2017). In reply—Defining physician burnout, and differentiating between burnout and depression. *Mayo Clinic Proceedings, 92*(9), 1456–1457. http://doi.org/10.1016/j.mayocp.2017.07.005

Niedhammer, I., Pineau, E., & Rosankis, E. (2024). The associations of psychosocial work exposures with suicidal ideation in the national French SUMER study. *Journal of Affective Disorders, 356*, 699–706. https://doi.org/10.1016/j.jad.2024.04.070

O'Connor, J. P., Stefic, E. C., & Gresock, C. J. (1957). Some patterns of depression. *Journal of Clinical Psychology, 13*, 122–125.

Orosz, A., Federspiel, A., Haisch, S., Seeher, C., Dierks, T., & Cattapan, K. (2017). A biological perspective on differences and similarities between burnout and depression. *Neuroscience & Biobehavioral Reviews, 73*, 112–122. https://doi.org/ 10.1016/j.neubiorev.2016.12.005

Pines, A., & Aronson, E. (1988). *Career burnout: Causes and cures*. The Free Press.

Pines, A., Aronson, E., & Kalfry, D. (1981). *Burnout: From tedium to personal growth*. The Free Press.

Pryce, C. R., Azzinnari, D., Spinelli, S., Seifritz, E., Tegethoff, M., & Meinlschmidt, G. (2011). Helplessness: A systematic translational review of theory and evidence for its relevance to understanding and treating depression. *Pharmacology & Therapeutics, 132*(3), 242–267. https://doi.org/10.1016/j.pharmthera.2011.06.006

Radloff, L. S. (1977). The CES-D scale: A self-report depression scale for research in the general population. *Applied Psychological Measurement, 1*(3), 385–401. https://doi.org/10.1177/014662167700100306

Reizer, A., & Mey-Raz, N. (2019). Slowing down vacation fade-out effects. *International Journal of Stress Management, 26*(3), 213–222. http://doi.org/10.1037/str0000103

Rönkkö, M., & Cho, E. (2022). An updated guideline for assessing discriminant validity. *Organizational Research Methods, 25*(1), 6–14. https://doi.org/10.1177/1094428120968614

Rosenthal, R. (1979). The file drawer problem and tolerance for null results. *Psychological Bulletin, 86*(3), 638–641. https://doi.org/10.1037/0033-2909.86.3.638

Rössler, W., Hengartner, M. P., Ajdacic-Gross, V., & Angst, J. (2015). Predictors of burnout: Results from a prospective community study. *European Archives of Psychiatry and Clinical Neuroscience, 265*(1), 19C25. https://doi.org/10.1007/s00406-014-0512-x

Rotenstein, L. S., Torre, M., Ramos, M. A., Rosales, R. C., Guille, C., Sen, S., & Mata, D. A. (2018). Prevalence of burnout among physicians: A systematic review. *Journal of the American Medical Association, 320*(11), 1131–1150. https://doi.org/10.1001/jama.2018.12777

Rothe, N., Steffen, J., Penz, M., Kirschbaum, C., & Walther, A. (2020). Examination of peripheral basal and reactive cortisol levels in major depressive disorder and the burnout syndrome: A systematic review. *Neuroscience & Biobehavioral Reviews, 114*, 232–270. https://doi.org/10.1016/j.neubiorev.2020.02.024

Schaufeli, W. B., & Buunk, B. P. (2004). Burnout: An overview of 25 years of research and theorizing. In M. J. Schabracq, J. A. M. Winnubst, & C. L. Cooper (Eds.), *The handbook of work and health psychology* (2nd ed.), (pp. 383–425). Wiley. https://doi.org/10.1002/0470013400.ch19

Schaufeli, W. B., Desart, S., & De Witte, H. (2020) Burnout Assessment Tool (BAT)—Development, validity, and reliability. *International Journal of Environmental Research and Public Health, 17*(24), 9495. https://doi.org/10.3390/ijerph17249495

Schaufeli, W. B., Leiter, M. P., & Maslach, C. (2009). Burnout: 35 years of research and practice. *Career Development International, 14*(3), 204–220. https://doi.org/10.1108/13620430910966406

Schonfeld, I. S. (2000). An updated look at depressive symptoms and job satisfaction in first-year women teachers. *Journal of Occupational and Organizational Psychology, 73*, 363–371. https://doi.org/10.1348/096317900167074

Schonfeld, I. S. (2006). School violence. In E. K. Kelloway, J. Barling, & J. J. Hurrell, Jr. (Eds.), *Handbook of workplace violence* (pp. 169–229). Sage Publications. https://doi.org/10.4135/9781412976947.n9

Schonfeld, I. S., & Bianchi, R. (2016). Burnout and depression: Two entities or one. *Journal of Clinical Psychology, 72*(1), 22–37. https://doi.org/10.1002/jclp.22229

Schonfeld, I. S., & Bianchi, R. (2021a). Psychiatrist burnout. *American Journal of Psychiatry, 178*(2), 204. https://doi.org/10.1176/appi.ajp.2020.20071110

Schonfeld, I. S., & Bianchi, R. (2021b). From burnout to occupational depression: Recent developments in research on job-related distress and occupational health. *Frontiers in Public Health, 9*(796401), 1–6. https://doi.org/10.3389/fpubh.2021.796401

Schonfeld, I. S., & Bianchi, R. (2022). Distress in the workplace: Characterizing the relationship of burnout measures to the Occupational Depression Inventory. *International Journal of Stress Management, 29*, 253–259. https://doi.org/10.1037/str0000261

Schonfeld, I. S., & Chang, C.-H. (2017). *Occupational health psychology: Work, stress, and health*. Springer Publishing Company. https://doi.org/10.1891/9780826199683

Schonfeld, I. S., & Farrell, E. (2010). Qualitative methods can enrich quantitative research on occupational stress: An example from one occupational group. In D. C. Ganster & P. L. Perrewé (Eds.), *Research in occupational stress and wellbeing series. Vol. 8. New developments in theoretical and conceptual approaches to job stress* (pp. 137–197). Bingley, UK: Emerald. https://doi.org/10.1108/S1479-3555(2010)0000008007

Schonfeld, I. S., & Santiago, E. A. (1994). Working conditions and psychological distress in first-year women teachers: Qualitative findings. In L. C. Blackman (Ed.), *What works? Synthesizing effective biomedical and psychosocial strategies for healthy families in the 21st century* (pp. 114–121). Indiana University School of Social Work.

Schonfeld, I. S., Bianchi, R., & Luehring-Jones, P. (2017). Consequences of job stress for the psychological well-being of teachers. In T. M. McIntyre, S. E. McIntyre, & D. J. Francis (Eds.), *Educator stress: An occupational health perspective* (pp. 55–75). Springer International Publishing. https://doi.org/10.1007/978-3-319-53053-6_3

Schonfeld, I. S., Verkuilen, J., & Bianchi, R. (2019a). Inquiry into the correlation between burnout and depression. *Journal of Occupational Health Psychology, 24*, 603–616. http://doi.org/10.1037/ocp0000151

Schonfeld, I. S., Verkuilen, J., & Bianchi, R. (2019b). An exploratory structural equation modeling bi-factor analytic approach to uncovering what burnout, depression, and anxiety scales measure. *Psychological Assessment, 31*, 1073–1079. http://doi.org/10.1037/pas0000721

Sen, S. (2022). Is it burnout or depression? Expanding efforts to improve physician well-being. *New England Journal of Medicine, 387*(18), 1629–1630. http://doi.org/10.1056/NEJMp2209540

Shirom, A., & Melamed, S. (2006). A comparison of the construct validity of two burnout measures in two groups of professionals. *International Journal of Stress Management, 13*, 176–200. http://doi.org/10.1037/1072-5245.13.2.176

Sinval, J., Vazquez, A., Hutz, C. S., Schaufeli, W. B., & Silva, S. (2022). Burnout assessment tool (BAT): Validity evidence from Brazil and Portugal. *International Journal of Environmental Research and Public Health, 19*(3), 1344. http://doi.org/10.3390/ijerph19031344

Sowden, J., Schonfeld, I. S., & Bianchi, R. (2022). Are Australian teachers burned-out or depressed? A confirmatory factor analytic study involving the Occupational Depression Inventory. *Journal of Psychosomatic Research, 157*, 110783. https://doi.org/10.1016/j.jpsychores.2022.110783

Spector, P. E. (2013). Survey design and measure development. In T. D. Little (Ed.), *The Oxford handbook of quantitative methods* (Vol. 1, pp. 170–188). Oxford University Press. https://doi.org/10.1093/oxfordhb/9780199934874.013.0009

Swingler, G., Verkuilen, J., Bianchi, R., & Schonfeld, I. S. (2023). Burnout and depression in teachers and members of other occupational groups: A systematic review and meta-analyses on potentially overlapping conditions. 15th International Conference on Work, Stress, and Health.

Terluin, B., Van Rhenen, W., Schaufeli, W. B., & De Haan, M. (2004). The Four-Dimensional Symptom Questionnaire (4DSQ): Measuring distress and other mental health problems in a working population. *Work & Stress, 18*(3), 187–207. https://doi.org/10.1080/0267837042000297535

Toker, S., Melamed, S., Berliner, S., Zeltser, D., & Shapira, I. (2012). Burnout and risk of coronary heart disease: A prospective study of 8838 employees. *Psychosomatic Medicine, 74*, 840–847. https://doi.org/10.1097/PSY.0b013e31826c3174

Verkuilen, J., Bianchi, R., Schonfeld, I. S., & Laurent, E. (2021). Burnout-depression overlap: Exploratory structural equation modeling bifactor analysis and network analysis. *Assessment, 28*(6), 1583–1600. https://doi.org/10.1177/1073191120911095

Westman, M., & Etzion, D. (2001). The impact of vacation and job stress on burnout and absenteeism. *Psychology and Health, 16*(5), 595–606. https://doi.org/10.1080/08870440108405529

Willner, P., Scheel-Kruger, J., & Belzung, C. (2013). The neurobiology of depression and antidepressant action. *Neuroscience & Biobehavioral Reviews, 37*(10), 2331–2371. https://doi.org/10.1016/j.neubiorev.2012.12.007

Wurm, W., Vogel, K., Holl, A., Ebner, C., Bayer, D., Mörkl, S., Szilagyi, I.-S., Hotter, E., Kapfhammer, H.-P., & Hofmann, P. (2016). Depression-burnout overlap in physicians. *PLoS One, 11*(3), Article e0149913. https://doi.org/10.1371/journal.pone.0149913

4

The Stigma Attached to Burnout

The term "stigma" (στίγμα) originates from the Greek verb "stízō" (στίζω), meaning "to prick" or "to tattoo" (Liddell et al., 1996). In ancient Greece, a stigma was a mark or brand, often created by pricking or burning the skin. Such marks were used to identify slaves, criminals, or others considered outcasts. However, they could also serve as positive symbols in religious, spiritual, and mystical contexts. The word was later adopted into Latin as "stigma," retaining essentially the same meaning. It is only in the sixteenth century that "stigma" entered the English language (*Oxford English Dictionary*, 2024). Over time, the figurative sense of the term, referring to a mark of disgrace or infamy, became increasingly prominent—this is the primary way the term is used today. This broader, metaphorical sense describes the societal rejection or condemnation associated with certain conditions, behaviors, or attributes, including mental illness (Gaebel et al., 2017).

In recent decades, stigma has garnered increasing attention in the organizational and clinical sciences (Brohan et al., 2012; Brouwers et al., 2020; Wheat et al., 2010), and researchers have refined the concept considerably. The stigma associated with mental illness is now held to involve several components, namely, stereotypes, prejudices, and discrimination (Sheehan et al., 2017). In addition, a distinction is commonly made between public stigma and self-stigma: "Public stigma refers to the negative attitudes held by members of the public about people with devalued characteristics. Self-stigma occurs when people internalize these public

Breaking Point: Job Stress, Occupational Depression, and the Myth of Burnout,
First Edition. Irvin Sam Schonfeld and Renzo Bianchi.
© 2025 John Wiley & Sons, Inc. Published 2025 by John Wiley & Sons, Inc.

attitudes and suffer numerous negative consequences as a result" (Corrigan & Rao, 2012, p. 464). Stigma is thought to have numerous harmful consequences, including delaying or preventing help-seeking and treatment (Henderson et al., 2013; McLaren et al., 2023; Oquendo et al., 2019). Not all types of stigma, however, appear to substantially influence such outcomes, calling for targeted antistigma actions and a cautious use of interventional resources (Schnyder et al., 2017; Yu et al., 2023). Stigma is generally understood as a dynamic phenomenon closely tied to the social practices and representations of a given population at a given moment in history. Across time and space, the same object can turn from nonstigmatized to stigmatized and vice versa.

Some Background Beliefs

Perhaps because the burnout construct emerged outside of the realm of psychiatry, from "a bottom-up and 'grass-roots' approach" to distress (Maslach et al., 2001, p. 398), the label of burnout has been assumed to convey little stigma (e.g., Schaufeli et al., 2009). This belief has been persistent, likely due to the ambiguous status of burnout (Oquendo et al., 2019). Indeed, though regarded as a health-threatening syndrome having clear medical relevance, burnout has never been formally classified nosologically and is not defined as a medical condition (World Health Organization, 2019). A corollary of the idea that burnout conveys little stigma is that the burnout label may allow working individuals to address their personal struggle with work-related distress more openly and more safely. Put differently, it may be easier to say, "I'm burned-out" than "I'm depressed," and less consequential to disclose a "burnout episode" than a "depressive episode" (Bahlmann et al., 2013; Oquendo et al., 2019). Burnout would thus function as a euphemism for conditions such as depression. By extension, if the stigma attached to burnout is minimal, that could help explain the popularity of the concept not only in the workforce but also within the research community. Regardless of whether one views the burnout construct as scientifically and clinically sound, it may at least serve the purpose of reducing stigma and encouraging individuals to seek care.

What Empirical Research Indicates

In recent years, empirical research on the stigma attached to burnout has grown. The findings that have accumulated reveal a tableau that belies the beliefs previously described. The available evidence suggests that the burnout label may be highly stigmatizing, making disclosure potentially harmful to affected individuals. Two studies, conducted by Sterkens and his colleagues, have been particularly helpful in advancing research on the stigma attached to the burnout label.

In the first of these two studies, Sterkens et al. (2021) investigated the hiring discrimination faced by candidates with a history of burnout. Using a vignette experiment, 425 Belgian recruiters from various industries were asked to evaluate fictitious job candidates. Each candidate's profile included a gap in employment history. The gap was attributed to one of four reasons: burnout, physical injury, personal reasons, or unemployment. The aim of the study was to assess how revealing a history of burnout influences recruiters' perceptions of the candidate's abilities and likelihood of being hired, compared to other reasons for employment gaps. The findings showed that candidates who disclosed a history of burnout were significantly less likely to be invited for a job interview or hired than those with gaps owing to other reasons. The recruiters' judgments were mainly driven by perceptions of lower stress tolerance and concerns about future absenteeism. Expectedly, the negative impact of revealing burnout was more pronounced for jobs requiring tolerance of high levels of stress. The authors concluded that burnout-related stigma plays a major role in hiring decisions, and addressing these biases could improve the reintegration of individuals recovering from burnout into the labor market.

In the second study, Sterkens et al. (2023) focused on job promotion. Using once again a vignette experiment and relying on more than 400 managers from the U.K. and United States, the study explored how burnout-related stigma influences managers' promotion decisions. Managers were asked to evaluate fictional candidates for internal promotions, with candidates varying in employment history (e.g., no interruptions, parental leave, sick leave following an accident, and stress-related leave due to burnout), tenure, performance, and other characteristics such as sex and age. The findings revealed that employees with a history of burnout were 34% less likely to be recommended for promotion compared to those without employment interruptions. The stigma associated with burnout primarily, and negatively, influenced the managers' perceptions of the employees' leadership capacity, stress tolerance, and ability to serve as role models. The stigma also negatively influenced the managers' estimates of the chances that the employees would find another job. Together, these perceptions explained almost half of the observed promotion decisions. Interestingly, female managers were found to impose a higher promotion penalty on candidates with a history of burnout compared to male managers. The study concluded that burnout stigma plays a significant role in promotion decisions, highlighting the challenges faced by employees recovering from burnout in advancing their careers.

These two studies suggest that a history of burnout can be a deterrent for recruiters in hiring and for managers in making promotion decisions. Far from being benign, the burnout label may thus need to be handled with caution in job contexts.

Burnout Versus Depression

It has been suggested that the success of the burnout construct may be related to the burnout label being less stigmatizing than the depression label (e.g., Oquendo et al., 2019). Several studies have compared the stigma attached to burnout and depression, tackling the issue from several different angles.

In a study conducted in Germany, Bahlmann et al. (2013) examined whether labeling a depressive episode as "burnout" instead of "depression" affected stigma and treatment recommendations. The researchers administered a stigma-related survey to representative samples of the German population in 2001 ($n = 5{,}024$) and again in 2011 ($n = 3{,}642$). Participants were presented with case vignettes describing individuals with depression, schizophrenia, or alcohol dependence. The vignettes did not include diagnostic labels, and participants were asked to describe what condition they believed the person had. The study found that labeling a depressive episode as "burnout" increased significantly between 2001 and 2011, from 0.3 to 10.2%. This trend was not observed for schizophrenia or alcohol dependence, which were rarely labeled as burnout. When participants used the term "burnout" to describe a depressive episode, they exhibited slightly less desire for social distance compared to when they used the label "depression." However, the label "burnout" was associated with fewer recommendations for professional treatments, such as psychotherapy, medication, or seeing a psychiatrist, than the label "depression." The main conclusion of the study was that while the term "burnout" may reduce social stigma compared to "depression," being identified as suffering from burnout may also result in fewer treatment recommendations, potentially leading to individuals with depressive disorders underutilizing treatment services. Thus, the increasing use of "burnout" as a label for depression may have both desirable and undesirable consequences for individuals suffering from mental health conditions.

In another German study, Mendel et al. (2015) investigated how different diagnostic labels affect managers' perceptions of employees' future job performance. The study presented to 748 managers vignettes depicting an employee with unspecific symptoms, such as sleep problems and social withdrawal, which could be indicative of various health conditions. Participants were randomly assigned to one of four groups. In each group, the vignettes labeled the employee's condition differently—burnout, depression, a private crisis, or hypothyroidism. The managers were then asked to evaluate the employee across eight dimensions, including the ability to work under pressure, the likelihood of future absences, the need for workplace assistance, and the level of trust in the employee's leadership potential. Mendel et al. hypothesized that burnout, which they considered less stigmatizing, would lead to more favorable evaluations than depression. However, the hypothesis was not supported. In fact, there was only one significant difference: Managers rated employees with depression more favorably than those with burnout in terms of ability to work under pressure. The findings suggested that burnout is not perceived more positively than depression and may even be associated with greater expectations of work-related impairment.

Nearly 10 years ago, we sought to compare the public stigma attached to burnout and depression and assess whether burnout and depression differ in their link to help-seeking attitudes and behaviors (Bianchi et al., 2016). To this end, we surveyed 1,046 schoolteachers employed in France. About half the teachers completed a survey about burnout, while the remaining participants completed a survey about depression. We found the burnout label to be slightly less stigmatizing than the depression label. However, the overall level of stigmatizing attitudes in our study sample turned out to be very small. Indeed, fewer than 1% of the participants in both the burnout-label and depression-label groups endorsed stigmatizing statements. Respondents considered burnout and depression similarly worth treating. In both the burnout-label group and the depression-label group, the extent of stigma respondents ascribed to burnout and depression was negatively correlated with the importance they assigned to consulting a clinician. Correlations were small to moderate in size. Finally, burnout and depression were associated with 12-month help-seeking behaviors and intentions to seek help to a similar extent when participants assessed their own levels of burnout and depression. All in all, no clear differences thus emerged in how burnout and depression were perceived.

Smith et al. (2023) further compared the perceptions of the burnout and depression labels in a survey of 676 Australians. Participants were asked to imagine that they were consulting with their general practitioner (GP) and were then presented with a scenario of the content of the consultation (there was a minor one-word difference in the scenarios presented to men and women). The scenario included a list of symptoms and a diagnosis provided by the GP at the end of the appointment. Participants were randomly assigned to one of four diagnostic label groups. The first group received a hypothetical scenario in which the doctor provided no diagnostic label for their reported symptoms (i.e., control group). For the second group, the doctor provided the diagnosis of "depression" to explain their symptoms. The third group received the diagnosis of "burnout" for their reported symptoms. The fourth and last group received a fictitious diagnostic label of "functional impairment syndrome." Only the diagnosis delivered differed across the conditions. Participants subsequently completed various outcome measures. The authors found that, although depression was perceived to be the most serious diagnostic label, there were no significant differences in the effect of the labels on help-seeking intention, self-stigma, worry, and attitudes toward the diagnosis. Interestingly, participants were more likely to envisage speaking about their condition with their boss in the depression-label group than in the burnout-label group. In sum, the study findings suggested that the burnout and depression labels had highly comparable stigma loads.

The authors concluded: "our results suggest that providing a burnout diagnosis to explain mild depressive symptoms in workplace/occupational contexts may not be more favorable in terms of alleviating stigma and increasing help-seeking" (pp. 80–81).

Studies that directly compared the effects of the burnout and depression labels allowed us to refine our understanding of the stigma surrounding burnout. Overall, what these studies suggest is not only that the burnout label carries stigma, but that the stigma attached to the burnout label is comparable to that of the depression label. It thus seems that the burnout label provides little benefit in terms of social acceptance owing to its non-medical origin.[1]

Destigmatizing Burnout

In attempting to mitigate burnout stigmatization, some researchers have advanced narratives emphasizing the role of external factors and downplaying that of internal factors in the development of burnout (e.g., Maslach & Leiter, 1997). Though likely driven by good intentions, such narratives tend to promote a victim mindset, potentially draining people of their sense of agency and control over adversity. Looking back on her own experience with burnout, Kempton (2024) described this type of narratives in the following terms: "there is no agency, as your circumstance is the result of others' actions; if someone else alone got you here, then only someone else can get you out." While the role of external factors (e.g., working conditions) in the etiology of job-related distress is undoubtedly important, it should not overshadow the implication of individual factors and reduce people to passive entities. Ironically enough, the promotion of a sense of helplessness and heteronomy is a path to depression.

On a different note, Sen (2022) aptly observed that efforts to avoid stigmatizing burnout have often come at the expense of stigmatizing other conditions—most notably, depression. In fact, burnout researchers have frequently used the idea of a burnout–depression distinction to destigmatize burnout, suggesting that, contrary to depression, burnout

---

1 It is unclear whether the burnout label has carried stigma from inception due to the relatively recent interest of researchers in the topic.

is not a result of individual weakness but the result of workplace problems (Epstein & Privitera, 2017; Maslach, 2017). Such messaging, aside from being based on a shaky distinction between burnout and depression (as per the evidence adduced in Chapter 3), mistakenly reduces depression to a person-level issue (Bianchi et al., 2017). The belief among some burnout researchers that depression is primarily an individual problem tells us a lot about how mental illness is perceived and conceived. In Chapter 1, however, we have described the critical role of unresolvable stress in the development of depression. The concern over stigma, loudly voiced by burnout researchers when burnout is in focus, seems to fade when the conversation turns to depression—or mental illness in general.

Conclusions

There is mounting evidence that the burnout label conveys considerable stigma. The stigmatizing character of burnout suggests that the label should not be used carelessly, especially in organizational settings. A history of burnout can be a barrier to both employment and job promotion. People identified as having experienced burnout are perceived as less able to cope with stressors and more fragile overall (e.g., more likely to be on sick leave [again]). Years ago, we had raised the possibility that, though scientifically and medically problematic, burnout may have some residual value as a euphemistic, low-stigma label for depression (Bianchi et al., 2016). This does not appear to be the case, further undermining burnout's utility.

The stigma attached to depression remains an unresolved issue (Bianchi et al., 2019; Gold et al., 2016; Pereira-Lima & Sen, 2024). There might be a few reasons to be optimistic, however. Depression is being demystified in the view of members of the public, with a growing understanding that virtually anyone can experience depression at some point if facing overwhelming life difficulties, including work-related difficulties (Angermeyer et al., 2013; Schomerus et al., 2022). Patients themselves make various inferences about the cause(s) of their depression, with work-related stress being one of the determinants most often invoked (Hansson et al., 2010; Read et al., 2015). These findings might signal that the stigma associated with depression is receding, possibly encouraging affected individuals to seek care and address the depressogenic factors in their lives.

As stakeholders, one of our responsibilities is to ensure that the therapeutic solutions we propose are demonstrably effective and adhere to the principle of *nonmaleficence*—the "do no harm" principle central to medicine. It is crucial that our solutions focus on individuals *and* their environment. Human beings can be viewed as both products and producers of their history, with the social world shaping individuals and individuals shaping the social world, in a virtually endless loop. If one gives any credit to this *coproduction view*, it becomes challenging to approach treatment without considering both internal and external factors.

References

Angermeyer, M. C., Millier, A., Rémuzat, C., Refaï, T., & Toumi, M. (2013). Attitudes and beliefs of the French public about schizophrenia and major depression: Results from a vignette-based population survey. *BMC Psychiatry*, *13*, 313. https://doi.org/10.1186/1471-244X-13-313

Bahlmann, J., Angermeyer, M. C., & Schomerus, G. (2013). "Burnout" statt "Depression"—eine Strategie zur Vermeidung von Stigma? [Calling it "burnout" instead of "depression"—a strategy to avoid stigma?]. *Psychiatrische Praxis*, *40*(2), 78–82. https://doi.org/10.1055/s-0032-1332891

Bianchi, R., Schonfeld, I. S., & Laurent, E. (2017). Burnout or depression: Both individual and social issue. *The Lancet*, *390*(10091), 230. https://doi.org/10.1016/S0140-6736(17)31606-9

Bianchi, R., Schonfeld, I. S., & Laurent, E. (2019). Burnout: Moving beyond the status quo. *International Journal of Stress Management*, *26*(1), 36–45. https://doi.org/10.1037/str0000088

Bianchi, R., Verkuilen, J., Brisson, R., Schonfeld, I. S., & Laurent, E. (2016). Burnout and depression: Label-related stigma, help-seeking, and syndrome overlap. *Psychiatry Research*, *245*, 91–98. https://doi.org/10.1016/j.psychres.2016.08.025

Brohan, E., Henderson, C., Wheat, K., Malcolm, E., Clement, S., Barley, E. A., Slade, M., & Thornicroft, G. (2012). Systematic review of beliefs, behaviours and influencing factors associated with disclosure of a mental health problem in the workplace. *BMC Psychiatry, 12*(1), 11. https://doi.org/10.1186/1471-244X-12-11

Brouwers, E. P. M., Joosen, M. C. W., van Zelst, C., & Van Weeghel, J. (2020). To disclose or not to disclose: A multi-stakeholder focus group study on mental health issues in the work environment. *Journal of Occupational Rehabilitation, 30*(1), 84–92. https://doi.org/10.1007/s10926-019-09848-z

Corrigan, P. W., & Rao, D. (2012). On the self-stigma of mental illness: Stages, disclosure, and strategies for change. *Canadian Journal of Psychiatry, 57*(8), 464–469. https://doi.org/10.1177/070674371205700804

Epstein, R. M., & Privitera, M. R. (2017). Physician burnout is better conceptualised as depression—Authors' reply. *The Lancet, 389*(10077), 1398. https://doi.org/10.1016/S0140-6736(17)30898-X

Gaebel, W., Rössler, W., & Sartorius, N. (2017). *The stigma of mental illness—End of the story?* Springer International Publishing/Springer Nature. https://doi.org/10.1007/978-3-319-27839-1

Gold, K. J., Andrew, L. B., Goldman, E. B., & Schwenk, T. L. (2016). "I would never want to have a mental health diagnosis on my record": A survey of female physicians on mental health diagnosis, treatment, and reporting. *General Hospital Psychiatry, 43*, 51–57. https://doi.org/https://doi.org/10.1016/j.genhosppsych.2016.09.004

Hansson, M., Chotai, J., & Bodlund, O. (2010). Patients' beliefs about the cause of their depression. *Journal of Affective Disorders, 124*(1), 54–59. https://doi.org/10.1016/j.jad.2009.10.032

Henderson, C., Evans-Lacko, S., & Thornicroft, G. (2013). Mental illness stigma, help seeking, and public health programs. *American Journal of Public Health, 103*(5), 777–780. https://doi.org/10.2105/AJPH.2012.301056

Kempton, C. L. (2024). Is a victim mindset perpetuating burnout in healthcare? *The American Journal of Medicine.* Advance online publication. https://doi.org/10.1016/j.amjmed.2024.08.023

Liddell, H. G., Scott, R., & Jones, H. S. (1996). *A Greek–English lexicon* (9th ed., with a revised supplement). Clarendon Press.

Maslach, C. (2017). Finding solutions to the problem of burnout. *Consulting Psychology Journal: Practice and Research, 69*(2), 143–152. https://doi.org/10.1037/cpb0000090

Maslach, C., & Leiter, M. P. (1997). *The truth about burnout: How organizations cause personal stress and what to do about it.* Jossey-Bass.

Maslach, C., Schaufeli, W. B., & Leiter, M. P. (2001). Job burnout. *Annual Review of Psychology*, *52*(1), 397–422. https://doi.org/10.1146/annurev.psych.52.1.397

McLaren, T., Peter, L.-J., Tomczyk, S., Muehlan, H., Schomerus, G., & Schmidt, S. (2023). The seeking mental health care model: Prediction of help-seeking for depressive symptoms by stigma and mental illness representations. *BMC Public Health*, *23*(1), 69. https://doi.org/10.1186/s12889-022-14937-5

Mendel, R., Kissling, W., Reichhart, T., Bühner, M., & Hamann, J. (2015). Managers' reactions towards employees' disclosure of psychiatric or somatic diagnoses. *Epidemiology and Psychiatric Sciences*, *24*(2), 146–149. https://doi.org/10.1017/S2045796013000711

Oquendo, M. A., Bernstein, C. A., & Mayer, L. E. S. (2019). A key differential diagnosis for physicians-major depression or burnout? *JAMA Psychiatry*, *76*(11), 1111–1112. https://doi.org/10.1001/jamapsychiatry.2019.1332

Oxford University Press. (2024). *Oxford English Dictionary*. Author.

Pereira-Lima, K., & Sen, S. (2024). Resident physician depression: Systemic challenges and possible solutions. *Trends in Molecular Medicine*. Advance online publication. https://doi.org/10.1016/j.molmed.2024.08.001

Read, J., Cartwright, C., Gibson, K., Shiels, C., & Magliano, L. (2015). Beliefs of people taking antidepressants about the causes of their own depression. *Journal of Affective Disorders*, *174*, 150–156. https://doi.org/10.1016/j.jad.2014.11.009

Schaufeli, W. B., Leiter, M. P., & Maslach, C. (2009). Burnout: 35 years of research and practice. *Career Development International*, *14*(3), 204–220. https://doi.org/10.1108/13620430910966406

Schnyder, N., Panczak, R., Groth, N., & Schultze-Lutter, F. (2017). Association between mental health-related stigma and active help-seeking: Systematic review and meta-analysis. *British Journal of Psychiatry*, *210*(4), 261–268. https://doi.org/10.1192/bjp.bp.116.189464

Schomerus, G., Schindler, S., Sander, C., Baumann, E., & Angermeyer, M. C. (2022). Changes in mental illness stigma over 30 years—improvement, persistence, or deterioration? *European Psychiatry*, *65*(1), e78. https://doi.org/10.1192/j.eurpsy.2022.2337

Sen, S. (2022). Is it burnout or depression? Expanding efforts to improve physician well-being. *New England Journal of Medicine*, *387*(18), 1629–1630. https://doi.org/10.1056/NEJMp2209540

Sheehan, L., Nieweglowski, K., & Corrigan, P. W. (2017). Structures and types of stigma. In W. Gaebel, W. Rössler, & N. Sartorius (Eds.), *The stigma of mental illness—End of the story?* (pp. 43–66). Springer International Publishing/Springer Nature. https://doi.org/10.1007/978-3-319-27839-1_3

Smith, J., Cvejic, E., Lal, T. J., Fisher, A., Tracy, M., & McCaffery, K. J. (2023). Impact of alternative terminology for depression on help-seeking intention: A randomized online trial. *Journal of Clinical Psychology, 79*(1), 68–85. https://doi.org/10.1002/jclp.23410

Sterkens, P., Baert, S., Rooman, C., & Derous, E. (2021). As if it weren't hard enough already: Breaking down hiring discrimination following burnout. *Economics & Human Biology, 43*, 101050. https://doi.org/10.1016/j.ehb.2021.101050

Sterkens, P., Baert, S., Rooman, C., & Derous, E. (2023). Why making promotion after a burnout is like boiling the ocean. *European Sociological Review, 39*(4), 516–531. https://doi.org/10.1093/esr/jcac055

Wheat, K., Brohan, E., Henderson, C., & Thornicroft, G. (2010). Mental illness and the workplace: Conceal or reveal? *Journal of the Royal Society of Medicine, 103*(3), 83–86. https://doi.org/10.1258/jrsm.2009.090317

World Health Organization. (2019, May 28). Burn-out an "occupational phenomenon": International Classification of Diseases. https://www.who.int/news/item/28-05-2019-burn-out-an-occupational-phenomenon-international-classification-of-diseases

Yu, B. C. L., Chio, F. H. N., Chan, K. K. Y., Mak, W. W. S., Zhang, G., Vogel, D., & Lai, M. H. C. (2023). Associations between public and self-stigma of help-seeking with help-seeking attitudes and intention: A meta-analytic structural equation modeling approach. *Journal of Counseling Psychology, 70*(1), 90–102. https://doi.org/10.1037/cou0000637

5

Interventions

The discipline within psychology with which the authors most closely identify is occupational health psychology (OHP). One of the tasks of OHP research is to develop measurement tools that validly assess psychosocial working conditions, work–family balance, safety climate, and work-related psychological symptoms (e.g., the Occupational Depression Inventory). OHP investigators also develop theories and test hypotheses generated by those theories. The hypotheses they test often bear on the relationship of working conditions to the mental and physical health and well-being of workers (Schonfeld & Chang, 2017). OHP researchers also develop interventions designed to enhance the health, safety, and well-being of workers. In this chapter, we are principally concerned with interventions that bear on depression, psychological distress, and burnout although these interventions can have broader effects (for example, on anxiety). Most interventions (treatments) are designed to help distressed individuals, whether their distress is work-related or not. These interventions were mainly developed by clinicians who are not associated with OHP.

Models of Interventions

We organized the interventions around a public health model (Cooper & Kompier, 1999; Schmidt, 1994). Within that model there are three general types of approaches to the prevention of illness: primary, secondary, and tertiary.

Breaking Point: Job Stress, Occupational Depression, and the Myth of Burnout,
First Edition. Irvin Sam Schonfeld and Renzo Bianchi.
© 2025 John Wiley & Sons, Inc. Published 2025 by John Wiley & Sons, Inc.

The purpose of a primary intervention is to prevent workplace stressors from developing in the first place or to remove those that currently exist, thereby preventing those stressors from affecting workers. In the workplace, primary interventions are often applied to all workers within an organizational unit or, sometimes, an entire organization. A primary intervention based on the demand–control model (see Chapter 1) would involve researchers, workers and their representatives (e.g., labor unions), and management collaborating to reorganize task structures in such a way that workers would be given more latitude over decisions pertaining to the tasks for which they are responsible. This type of intervention is related to the idea that increased latitude has a positive effect on workers' mental and physical health as well as their general well-being (Schonfeld & Chang, 2017).

Some workers, however, are already at risk for health problems and injuries although the problems are not full-blown. A secondary intervention targets that subset of workers. It involves early detection and early treatment before a health problem can become disabling (Joyce et al., 2016). A program designed to help healthy workers who smoke to quit is an example of a secondary intervention. The program may provide once- or twice-weekly workshops, run by health educators, that are designed to help those workers reduce cigarette consumption and, eventually, quit.

Another example of a secondary intervention involves targeting workers who have experienced the beginnings of an elevation in depressive symptoms. In this example, a coworker has started to direct, at first "playfully," derisive remarks at a target worker (e.g., making fun of the target worker's haircut or clothing). The intervention would involve an OHP specialist working with the human resources or employee assistance department to first conduct an anonymous survey designed to find out if any workers have experienced untoward problems such as bullying. The survey includes an invitation to workers who have experienced work-related problems to speak privately and candidly with the specialist. The worker who has been the target of the coworker completes the survey and takes up the invitation to go to the office to discuss these difficulties. Concerned for the well-being of the worker, the OHP specialist then takes steps to put a stop to the offensive behaviors before they escalate in seriousness and harm the victim further. An effective specialist would also have the sensitivity to respect the feelings of a perpetrator who may be unaware of the extent of harm done. Goals of the OHP specialist include improving relationships among coworkers and reducing tensions.

Tertiary interventions are directed at those workers who have already experienced significant declines in mental or physical health. These interventions, which typically are individually based, are designed to help already-affected workers recover. An organization may provide workers who are clinically depressed access to a clinical psychologist or psychiatrist for treatment. Some workers may seek treatment independently of the organization in order to protect their privacy and/or prevent negative repercussions of their condition from affecting their job status.

Richardson and Rothstein (2008) noted that the success of interventions can be assessed at several different levels. Success can be assessed at the organizational level (e.g., reductions in absenteeism, increased productivity). The success of interventions can also be assessed at the individual psychological level (e.g., reductions in depressive or burnout symptoms in workers) or physiological level (e.g., reductions in blood pressure in workers). The principal focus of this chapter, however, is the impact of interventions on depressive and burnout symptoms.

In discussing interventions later in the chapter, we work backward from tertiary to primary interventions. We note that most research on depressive conditions has involved tertiary interventions. We limit ourselves here to discussions of each of two important tertiary psychotherapeutic treatments, namely cognitive behavioral therapy (CBT) and interpersonal therapy (IPT), although we devote some coverage to behavioral activation and mindfulness therapies because of their connection to CBT.

CBT and IPT are the most researched types of psychotherapeutic treatments for depression (Cuijpers et al., 2023a). We will discuss the meta-analytic evidence derived from the many experiments that bear on CBT and IPT. We believe that our focus on CBT and IPT will be instructive regarding the major currents in research on tertiary psychotherapeutic interventions. Research on tertiary treatments for burnout have been scarcer. We will *not* review the variety of pharmacotherapies (antidepressant treatments) although we will examine research that looks at the combination of psychotherapy and pharmacotherapy.

After the section on tertiary interventions, we cover primary and secondary interventions together because the dividing line between them in the context of approaches to reducing work-related distress and burnout is porous. The relevant meta-analyses tend to group those interventions together.

Randomized Control Trials and Meta-analyses

Because intervention research and the application of meta-analyses to such research may be unfamiliar to nonspecialists, we wrote this brief section to help nonspecialist readers better understand the material that follows. A reader who has research experience may want to skip the section.

Randomized controlled trials (RCTs) help us understand the impact of a treatment such as CBT on depression or burnout. An RCT is an experiment. It comprises experimental (treatment) and control groups. Although no single study can conclusively establish a cause–effect relationship, the RCT is considered the gold standard in terms of helping researchers infer cause–effect relations in biomedical and psychological/psychiatric treatment research. As RCTs demonstrating the success of a particular type of treatment get replicated, confidence in the efficacy of the treatment grows. The RCT involves randomly assigning (many researchers use the term "allocating") members of the pool of research participants, sometimes called the "experimental units," to experimental and control groups (Schonfeld & Chang, 2017). With random allocation every participant has the same probability of being assigned to the treatment or control group (for ease of exposition, we limit ourselves to two groups, but RCTs can involve more than two treatment and/or control groups). Random assignment to groups ensures, particularly when sample size is large, that members of the treatment and control groups will, on average, be similar on most characteristics, including characteristics that were measured before the treatment starts (e.g., years of schooling) and even characteristics that were not measured or could not be measured (e.g., a grandparent's health history). Ideally, members of the treatment and control groups would be similar on all characteristics, except one, that one characteristic being group membership.

Sometimes it is impractical for the organizations that host researchers to allow the investigators to randomize individuals into treatment and control groups. This situation particularly applies to the case in primary interventions. In that case, researchers conduct cluster RCTs (cRCTs). The experimental units that get randomized are clusters of individuals such as organizational units or entire organizations. For example, Lucas et al. (2012) randomly allocated blocks of physicians to rotations of different lengths to understand the impact of rotation length on burnout. Even though clusters of physicians got randomly allocated to different treatments, the study is still an experiment. The previously mentioned study by Lucas et al. is part of the assemblage of studies in Panagioti et al.'s (2017) meta-analysis. In a study we look at in more detail later, Kossek et al. (2019) randomly assigned entire organizations to treatment and control conditions.

The treatment in a tertiary intervention study would ordinarily be a form of psychotherapy such as CBT or IPT, or pharmacotherapy. The control condition could be a waiting list that lasts about as long as the therapy, "treatment as usual" with a general practitioner, a placebo, and so forth. Ideally, assessments of the symptoms in the participants would take place before study participants are randomized into groups (pre-test) and after the treatment phase has been completed (post-test). Many RCTs also assess symptoms 6 and/or 12 months after the treatment has been completed (long-term follow-up).

To minimize the risk of biasing results, assessments of the participants would be "masked." In other words, observers who assess the symptoms and everyday functioning of participants are blinded to whether a participant was assigned to the experimental (treatment) or control condition. RCTs involving drug and placebo conditions are often "double-blind," that is, both the observers *and* the participants are not permitted to know the group to which the participants were assigned. Of course, in psychotherapy efficacy research it is basically impossible to mask group membership from the participants.

In addition, some research teams studying the efficacy of a treatment employ a conservative, "intention-to-treat" paradigm (Riegelman, 2005). In this paradigm, participants who don't strictly follow the intervention plan or stop taking the drug (or placebo) are nevertheless included in the study results. The research design thus addresses the question of whether *prescribing* the intervention leads to a different outcome than prescribing the control condition. The intention-to-treat paradigm in some sense mirrors what happens in life when individuals seek treatment from healthcare professionals; patients conform to the treatment plan to varying degrees. Kossek et al. (2019) in evaluating the impact of an intervention aimed at reducing psychological symptoms and life stress used an intention-to-treat approach. As a supplemental analysis, some investigators (not Kossek et al.) who employ an intention-to-treat approach also conduct an "as-treated" analysis that excludes participants who sharply deviated from the study protocol.

RCTs have inclusion and exclusion criteria regarding who can participate. An RCT in a psychotherapy efficacy study would have strict inclusion criteria. An example of an inclusion criterion would be a person having been diagnosed for major depressive disorder or having a score on a psychological symptom scale (e.g., the Hamilton Rating Scale for Depression) that is above a predetermined symptom threshold marking significant dysphoric feelings. RCTs also have strict exclusion criteria. For example, an RCT designed to assess a treatment for depression is likely to exclude individuals whose depression is secondary to alcohol abuse (which a clinician would treat differently).

Meta-analyses, which we cover later in the chapter, are likely to include RCTs, i.e. true experiments, and exclude quasi-experiments. A quasi-experiment has treatment and control groups like an RCT; research participants, however, are not randomly assigned to the groups. The research typically proceeds with the treatment and control conditions applied to pre-existing groups. Without random allocation of participants to treatment and control groups, a *sine qua non* for RCTs, it is questionable that the groups will be similar on most background characteristics.

As mentioned earlier, no one RCT can demonstrate the efficacy needed to ensure confidence that a particular treatment can help individuals suffering from, say, depression. Confidence in a type of treatment increases when many RCTs support the treatment's efficacy. This is where meta-analyses come into play.

Meta-analyses that bear on RCTs differ from the type of meta-analyses we described in in earlier chapters, which apply to correlation and regression coefficients in nonexperimental research (e.g., cross-sectional and longitudinal studies). In RCT-related meta-analyses, researchers target high-quality randomized treatment–control experiments. One potential obstacle to averaging the results of RCTs is that they use a variety of different measures of an outcome such as depressive symptoms to assess the impact of treatments in comparison to control conditions, ostensibly making the results of the studies incommensurable. For example, some studies assess outcomes by using the Hamilton Rating Scale for Depression, other studies use the Beck Depression Inventory, others use the PHQ-9, and so on.

In meta-analyses, there are ways of making the results of RCTs more or less commensurate. Meta-analysts often compare the treatment and control groups by calculating a statistic they derive from results from each relevant RCT-related publication. That statistic is Cohen's d (Cohen, 1988). In an example from an RCT involving a treatment for depressive symptoms, Cohen's d would involve calculating the difference between (1) the mean of the post-treatment depressive symptom scores of the participants in the treatment group and (2) the mean of the contemporaneous scores of the control group; then that difference is divided by the pooled standard deviation[1]:

$$d = [Mean_{Treatment} - Mean_{Control}] / s_{Pooled}$$

Cohen established a rule of thumb outlining what could be considered small ($d = .20$), medium ($d = .50$), and large ($d = .80$) effect sizes. Like the correlation coefficient, Cohen's d provides a common metric for comparing and averaging the results of studies. Cohen's d enables researchers to calculate an average of the effects of all the RCTs devoted to a specific treatment, like CBT. Thus, Cohen's d is a measure of *effect size*. A comparable measure of effect size is Hedges's g. Hedges's g can be interpreted like Cohen's d, although it is more complicated computationally. Hedges's g is particularly useful when sample size is small; Cohen's d has an upward bias in small samples (Hedges & Olkin, 1985). In the meta-analyses described later, some researchers employed Hedges's g and others, Cohen's d.

As mentioned in a footnote in Chapter 2, there are fixed- and random-effects meta-analyses, and these have implications for meta-analyses involving RCTs as well as correlational and regression-based studies (Borenstein et al., 2021; Dettori et al., 2022). The fixed-effects model assumes that one "true" effect size underlies much of the variation

---

[1] The standard deviation, s, is a statistic that indexes the dispersion of a group's scores around the group's mean. The pooled standard deviation, s_{pooled}, is a weighted average (weighted by the size of each group) of the standard deviations in the treatment and control groups.

in the effects in the primary studies that have been assembled for a meta-analysis. Variation in the primary studies' effect sizes is assumed to reflect sampling error. In the fixed-effects model, meta-analysts average the RCTs' effect sizes, with each RCT's effect size weighted by its sample size. The goal is to estimate the "true" effect size.

Unlike in the fixed-effects model, in the random-effects model, true effects themselves are assumed to vary among the primary RCTs. As in fixed-effects models, sampling error also contributes to variation among the RCTs' effect sizes. Thus, there are two sources of variation in the random-effects model, sampling error *and* study-to-study variation in the true effects. The goal of the random-effects meta-analysis is to estimate the mean effect size, not the one "true" effect size.

In the random-effects model the effect sizes are assumed to be a random sample of all the possible effect sizes, which has consequences for how the weighted average of the RCTs' effect sizes is calculated. In the random-effects model, large RCTs have larger weights but those weights would be *smaller* than the weights that would be found if the RCTs were part of a fixed-effects meta-analysis. Small RCTs have smaller weights, but those weights would be *larger* than the weights that would be found if the RCTs were part of a fixed-effects meta-analysis. Borenstein et al. (2021) wrote that in the random effects meta-analysis "we cannot discount a small study by giving it a very small weight (the way we would in a fixed-effect analysis) . . . By the same logic we cannot give too much weight to a very large study (the way we might in a fixed-effect analysis). Our goal is to estimate the mean effect in a range of studies, and we do not want that overall estimate to be overly influenced by any one of them" (pp. 72–73). In all the meta-analyses we cover in this chapter, the researchers used the generally more conservative random-effects models.

The *file drawer problem* is a challenge that can affect the confidence we have in the results of some of the meta-analyses described in the section on primary and secondary interventions. The file drawer problem, first described in print by Robert Rosenthal (1979), acknowledges that investigators are more likely to publish results that are consistent with their hypotheses and refrain from publishing results that are not. That tendency can handicap meta-analyses that are based on published studies. One way to address the problem is to include unpublished studies such as dissertations in a meta-analysis. A number of researchers have included unpublished studies in the meta-analyses described later (e.g., Richardson & Rothstein, 2008). Even if researchers include all published studies and dissertations, what about the studies that were conducted that were never released but that show that an intervention failed to reduce the symptom levels of participants in intervention groups or even unintentionally worsened their symptom levels?

Another way to address the file drawer problem is to calculate the "fail-safe N" (Orwin, 1983; Rosenthal, 1979). Conceptually, the fail-safe N is an estimate of the number of relevant but missing RCTs "averaging null results" (Rosenthal, 1979) that investigators would have had to file away and, by virtue of having been filed away, would make the average effect of the RCTs in a meta-analysis statistically significant. If the number of filed-away RCTs needed to reduce a significant effect found in a meta-analysis to nonsignificance is unrealistically large, we would be more likely to accept the results of the meta-analysis. The file drawer problem is particularly important to our discussion of the meta-analyses conducted for the primary and secondary intervention studies, where meta-analyses with fewer than ten RCTs abound. Fortunately, the numbers of tertiary intervention RCTs in several meta-analyses are large, where $k > 50$, k being the symbol for the number of RCTs. Large ks make it unlikely that many null RCT results were put in file drawers around the world, especially given the amount of work and the sizes of the teams required to mount such studies.

Tertiary Interventions

Psychotherapy is a tertiary intervention. According to the *APA Dictionary of Psychology* (VandenBos, 2015), psychotherapy is "any psychological service provided by a trained professional that primarily uses forms of communication and interaction to assess, diagnose, and treat dysfunctional emotional reactions, ways of thinking, and behavior patterns" (p. 863). It is a "talk therapy" practiced by a licensed psychotherapist who has undergone training to treat mental health problems such as depression. Although cognitive behavioral therapy and interpersonal therapy are talk therapies, they also promote patients getting involved in activities in their social environments. The therapist can be a clinical psychologist, psychiatrist, mental health counselor, psychiatric nurse, or clinical social worker.

Tertiary interventions involve individuals who have already developed a psychiatric or medical disorder. Tertiary interventions in psychiatry and psychology have been subject to considerably more research than primary and secondary interventions. Psychology and psychiatry have made significant progress in developing psychotherapeutic treatments designed to help individuals suffering from high levels of depressive symptoms and have employed RCTs to assess the efficacy of those treatments in improving the mental health of patients. Sometimes psychotherapies have been used to treat burnout; however, the number of RCTs pertaining to the efficacy of psychotherapies in treating burnout is small compared to the number of RCTs that assess the efficacy of psychotherapeutic treatments for depression. We note that it is rare that tertiary psychotherapeutic treatments have been tailored to psychological symptoms that are specifically work-related and that have been tested by way of RCTs (Schramm et al., 2020). The psychotherapeutic interventions we describe have been developed to deal with depressogenic problems wherever they occur—inside and outside of work. In some organizations, care management personnel screen current workers for depression. Such personnel reach out to depressed employees to recommend that these employees seek outpatient treatment such as psychotherapy (Joyce et al., 2016).

Cognitive behavioral therapy (CBT) is by far the most researched evidence-based psychotherapeutic treatment for depression. The efficacy of CBT has been the subject of more RCTs than any other form of psychotherapy (Cuijpers et al., 2023a). CBT originated with Aaron T. Beck and was influenced by Albert Ellis (Kellogg & Young, 2008), both of whom we described in Chapter 1. In what was originally a psychoanalytic practice, Beck (1997) observed that the largely negative "automatic thoughts" of his depressed patients tended to lead to unfortunate consequences for their well-being. In response, he was motivated to develop a "cognitive therapy" (Beck, 1997). Although Beck originally developed cognitive therapy to treat depression, he and others later expanded the therapy to treat other disorders. Despite its name, cognitive therapy involves behavioral techniques—for example, social skills training—pioneered by such figures as B. F. Skinner.

Cognitive therapy evolved into CBT (Kellogg & Young, 2008). In the CBT framework, mental disorders are believed to result from maladaptive thinking. A goal of CBT, which is mainly a short-term therapy that often lasts less than a year (and often less than 6 months), is to change the thinking of depressed patients, with the idea that emotional change will follow. According to Beck, a "cognitive triad" is the core of depression. The cognitive triad refers to negative thoughts depressed individuals hold about their self-worth, the world, and their personal future (Beck, 1997; Craighead et al., 2015). In Beck's view, as patients' thinking changes with the help of CBT and becomes more rational, the depression lifts and they are better able to take control of their mood.

With the help of the CBT-oriented clinician, patients evaluate the reasonableness of their thoughts and feelings. Are there logical errors in the person's thinking? Does the individual overgeneralize feelings of failure when a negative event or setback occurs at work? Does the individual magnify the implications of a minor hindrance? Does the individual need help in learning to be more assertive in situations involving a difficult coworker? Do patients minimize the value of their job-related accomplishments?

The therapy is present-focused. Unlike classical psychoanalysis, CBT is not centered on exhuming memories from childhood. The therapy includes helping patients adopt strategies that are organized to increase their activities out in the world, thus underlining the cognitive *behavioral* nature of the therapy. During those activities, patients are encouraged to monitor their thoughts and feelings.

As the therapy progresses, the patient's system of beliefs comes into focus. As the mental health of the patient improves, the clinician helps the patient develop strategies to combat inclinations toward the negative thinking that could foreshadow another episode of depression or different mental health problems. Such an approach is thought to reduce the risk of relapse.

Newer forms of CBT have added acceptance and commitment components. The acceptance component involves encouraging patients to stop trying to avoid negative thoughts and feelings, but rather to accept them without letting them prevent patients from pursuing valued life goals (Hayes et al., 2006). Acceptance in CBT emphasizes "mindfulness, emotions, acceptance, the relationship of the clients to their own experiences, values, goals, and meta-cognition"[2] (Li et al., 2024, p. 106).

---

2 Meta-cognition refers to individuals' awareness of their own thought processes; patients can harness that awareness to better control their thoughts and behavior.

The commitment component to this new approach to CBT involves the therapist encouraging the patient (through skills training, real-world practice, and other techniques) to adopt patterns of action based on the patient's short-, medium-, and long-term goals (Hayes et al., 2006). CBT with acceptance and commitment therapy (ACT) components has been used in treating job-related burnout (Prudenzi et al., 2021). Prudenzi et al.'s meta-analysis of the efficacy of group-formatted ACT treatments ($k = 9$) on work-related distress (assessed with mostly burnout measures but also with some other work-related symptom scales) found no statistically significant advantage for the ACT intervention over the control conditions at post-test; they did, however, find a small significant effect favoring ACT ($k = 8$) at later follow-up periods ($g = -0.30$).

Meta-analytic evidence consistently demonstrates the beneficial effects of CBT for individuals suffering from depression. In a meta-analysis (Cuijpers et al., 2013) that involved 95 RCT-driven comparisons against a control condition (e.g., wait list; care as usual), CBT showed a large and significant reduction in depressive symptoms ($g = -0.71$), although when limited to higher-quality studies, the effect size was moderate ($g = -0.53$). Other supporting evidence for the efficacy of CBT comes from Ljótsson et al.'s (2015) large ($k = 70$) meta-analysis.

Apropos of the evidence showing that CBT is effective in treating depression, we also note large-scale ($k = 522$) meta-analytic evidence, based on remission rates,[3] from RCTs that demonstrate that antidepressant medications can be helpful in treating individuals suffering from depression (Cipriani et al., 2018). In a comparison of CBT to pharmacotherapy based on 20 RCTs, there was no significant difference in efficacy (Cuijpers et al., 2013). In a limited number of comparisons ($3 < k < 16$) with other psychotherapies, the research team found CBT to be no more effective in reducing symptom levels. In a meta-analysis to be described in more detail later, Cuijpers et al. (2020) found that CBT and pharmacotherapy were about equally effective in helping depressed individuals. The research team also found that initial depression severity does not moderate the efficacy of CBT versus pharmacotherapy or CBT versus placebo pill. The finding bearing on depression severity echoed

---

3 The remission rates were reflected in odds ratios (see Chapter 2) rather than in terms of d and g.

the results of an earlier five-sample meta-analysis pitting CBT against placebo pill control conditions (Furukawa et al., 2017).

Ijaz et al. (2018) conducted a small meta-analysis involving individuals who were suffering from treatment-resistant depression, that is, depression the intensity of which does not lessen with antidepressant treatment. Based on the pooling of three RCTs in which antidepressants combined with CBT were compared to antidepressants alone, the research team found improved remission for the group getting the combined treatment and a reduction in symptoms ($d \approx -0.30$) beyond what the individual antidepressants alone provide. A limitation of the meta-analysis is that the results are based on only three RCTs with one with a very large sample dominating the findings.

One recent massive meta-analysis (Li et al., 2024) assembled 341 RCTs bearing on the impact of CBT on depression in China ($k = 34$) and the rest of the world ($k = 307$). The average effect size in Chinese samples was very large ($g = -1.19$). The average effect size in the rest of the world was also large ($g = -0.82$) but significantly smaller than the effect in China.

In connection to CBT and work, Xu et al. (2024) conducted meta-analyses involving tertiary RCTs that comprised employees who took a sick leave or were on a sick leave resulting from an incident at work. Sick leave was defined as taking more than 60 consecutive days off from work or taking three months off from work over 12 months. Some studies concerned depression. Still others concerned musculoskeletal (MSK) problems. CBT delivered face to face ($k = 12$) was found to significantly reduce the length of sick leave by an average of 8.7 days and CBT delivered remotely ($k = 3$), an average of 13.5 days. Averaging effect sizes, CBT was significantly more effective than the control conditions in reducing depressive symptoms, although the effect size was small ($d,g = -0.18$).[4]

Some investigators have conducted research on the impact of vacations on worker burnout. The research findings indicate short-term postvacation relief; however, a fade-out of beneficial vacation-related effects occurs between two weeks and one month (Kühnel & Sonnentag, 2011; Westman & Eden, 1997; Westman & Etzion, 2001). These results are not surprising because vacations do not address the stressors that may

---

4 It was not clear if the authors used Cohen's *d* or Hedges's *g*.

cause burnout or the worker's thoughts, perceptions, and social behaviors relevant to conditions at the workplace. Individuals who have experienced burnout have been treated with CBT and mindfulness-based cognitive therapy (which is discussed a little later). A meta-analysis (Ren et al., 2019) examined CBT and CBT with an acceptance-and-commitment component in connection to burnout, among other outcomes. The investigators, however, mixed together burnout and many other outcomes (e.g., depression, anxiety, pain, substance abuse), not permitting a clear understanding of the impact of CBT on burnout.

Behavioral activation (BA) is one aspect of CBT. In terms of BA, CBT-oriented psychotherapists, consistent with BA theory, encourage depressed patients to have positive, rewarding (reinforcing) interactions with their environment and desist from interacting with aspects of their environment that are depressogenic. BA is also a type of psychotherapy. Although related to CBT, BA has roots in Peter Lewinsohn's behavioral model for treating depression and can stand somewhat apart from CBT. In itself, BA is "a structured, brief psychotherapeutic approach that aims to (a) increase engagement in adaptive activities (which often are those associated with the experience of pleasure or mastery), (b) decrease engagement in activities that maintain depression or increase risk for depression, and (c) solve problems that limit access to reward or that maintain or increase aversive control" (Dimidjian et al., 2011, pp. 3–4). Cuijpers et al. (2023b) conducted a meta-analysis of 22 RCTs that encompassed BA treatments for depression but were *not* components of CBT. When they limited the meta-analysis to RCTs with low risk of bias ($k = 9$), they found a medium effect for symptom reduction ($g = -0.56$).[5]

Mindfulness therapy, which was mentioned previously, is a cognitive intervention. It is rooted in Buddhist mindfulness meditation (Grossman, 2015; Virgili, 2015). Mindfulness involves the quiet, purposeful, and nonjudgmental paying of attention to what is going on in the present moment (Sekhar et al., 2021). The therapy is often called *mindfulness-based cognitive therapy* or, in the workplace, *mindfulness-based stress reduction*. The therapy includes enhancing a person's ability to be conscious of the here and now, including internal states such as emotions, physical

---

5 The research team did not include a negative sign for reduced symptoms but to be consistent with our reporting, we included it here and elsewhere.

sensations, cognitions, and (harmful) habitual responses. It involves "moment-to-moment attention to perceptible experience" (Grossman, 2015). Other features of the therapy include the development of increased patience with and acceptance of one's experience. The therapy is often conducted in a series of 2- to 2-and-a-half-hour group sessions over the course of eight weeks or a daylong retreat (Bartlett et al., 2019; Virgili, 2015). Meta-analyses sometimes group mindfulness treatments, because of their meditation component, with interventions that involve relaxation (Estevez Cores et al., 2021).

The evidence from a meta-analysis (Bartlett et al., 2019) involving eight RCTs shows that the mindfulness treatments led to statistically significant post-treatment declines in depressive symptoms; the effect, however, was reduced to nonsignificance when publication bias was controlled. Barlett et al. identified only four studies that addressed EE and three apiece that addressed DP and PA; no significant effects were observed. Another meta-analysis (Sekhar et al., 2021) found no significant post-test effect for RCTs assessing the influence of mindfulness on depression ($k = 4$) and burnout ($k = 3$) in medical students and junior doctors. Miao et al. (2023) in their meta-analysis ($k = 9$) found a significant medium effect ($d = -0.53$) for mindfulness treatments in reducing depressive symptoms in MDD patients. A meta-analysis (Haslam et al., 2023) that concerned tertiary treatments, for example, mindfulness and coaching but neither CBT nor interpersonal therapy (see subsequent discussion), for burnout in physicians involved 38 weak RCTs (e.g., investigators not blinded). The research team did not find clinically meaningful differences between the treatment and control conditions.

Interpersonal therapy (IPT) is, like CBT, an evidence-based, present-focused psychotherapy that has been used to treat depression. IPT was codeveloped by Gerald L. Klerman and Myrna M. Weissman for the purpose of helping individuals recover from depression (Weissman et al., 2018). Like CBT, the therapy often lasts less than a year (often less than 4 months). Klerman and Weissman were influenced by the work of Adolf Meyer (see Chapter 1) and Harry Stack Sullivan (1953); both regarded interpersonal relationships as important influences on the development and course of psychiatric disorder (Markowitz & Weissman, 2012). IPT is thus based on the idea that the social/interpersonal context of a person's life is important to the development and maintenance of depression. Episodes of depression are often connected to the experience of stressful interpersonal events, an idea that recalls the discussion in Chapter 1 of the research of Brown and Harris and their book *The Social Origins of Depression*.

Clinicians can use their understanding of that interpersonal context to help the patient recognize the role of interpersonal factors in sustaining depressive symptoms and guide the patient to recovery (Weissman et al., 2018). The interpersonal context can include such difficulties as an intense role-related dispute at work or the break-up of a romantic relationship. Depressed individuals often blame themselves for work or other problems although the sources of those problems are usually more complicated. An important ingredient in IPT is the patient's learning social skills that will help in resolving many stressful interpersonal situations and build good relationships with others at work and outside of work. Good relationships are important to a person's mental health.

The therapist frames an episode of depression as a "treatable medical condition that was not the patient's fault" (Markowitz & Weissman, 2012). In addition, the therapist allows patients to validate anger associated with social situations, but in a socially appropriate manner. The therapist also encourages patients to engage more fully with their social environment. Because the therapy is time-limited, there is mild pressure on patients to learn to assert themselves in the immediate social environment. The goal of the assertiveness training is to ensure that patients can meet their needs. Socially appropriate risk-taking is also encouraged. The therapist provides reinforcement for social successes. As the therapy winds down, the therapist and patient review the patient's accomplishments. It is, however, possible for the individual to return for occasional sessions for maintenance purposes after the therapy has concluded.

In a meta-analysis involving 31 RCTs (Cuijpers et al., 2016), IPT was found to have a medium effect ($g = -0.60$) in helping individuals during acute-phase depression. When compared to antidepressant medication, there was no significant difference in efficacy. In an innovative meta-analysis involving 101 RCTs aimed mainly at individuals with moderate levels of depressive symptoms, Cuijpers et al. (2020) found that CBT, IPT, and antidepressant treatment were about equally better than control conditions in terms of remission. They, however, found that the combination of psychotherapy and pharmacotherapy had improved remission (~25%) better than what any of the therapies could do alone and reduced depressive symptom levels better than what pharmacotherapy could do alone

($d = -0.37$) and better than what psychotherapy could do alone ($d = -0.15$). The researchers noted, however, that most patients, to avoid side effects of antidepressant medication, find psychotherapy more acceptable than pharmacotherapy.

In the absence of meta-analyses bearing on the impact of IPT on job-related burnout, we found only one small RCT involving workers at a long-term care facility ($n = 50$) (Oral & Karakurt, 2024). IPT's impact in reducing symptoms of emotional exhaustion was large ($d = -1.11$). Apropos of other IPT-related tertiary interventions specifically bearing on work-related mental health problems, we identified Schramm et al.'s (2020) even smaller ($n = 26$) RCT. In this study, IPT had a large effect on symptom reduction in outpatients with work-related depression ($d = -0.79$).

Thoughts on IPT and CBT

Considering the growing number of psychotherapy efficacy studies on depression, Cuijpers et al. (2023a) identified 562 studies containing 669 RCTs that compared treatment and control conditions. The average effect size across all the psychotherapies was between medium and large ($g = -0.67$). The average effect size for CBT was large ($g = -0.73$; $k = 347$) and the average effect size for IPT, medium ($g = -0.43$; $k = 51$). The evidence indicates that a person experiencing high levels of depressive symptoms can benefit from either CBT or IPT. Although not the subject of this book, but as a matter of public interest, we note that the results bearing on the effectiveness of psychotherapy apply not just to adults but to children and adolescents as well.

In summary, the research is compelling in indicating that the tertiary CBT and IPT psychotherapy interventions, when implemented by trained professionals, can help individuals suffering from high levels of depressive symptoms. Many of the studies reviewed had varying follow-up periods after therapy concluded. Cuijpers et al. (2019) found that differences favoring symptom reduction in the intervention groups versus care-as-usual controls ($k = 19$; see Appendix K) showed evidence of long-term effectiveness. We note that by the numbers, research on psychotherapy efficacy has included more female than male participants; the evidence, however, indicates, at least for CBT (and pharmacotherapy), an absence of intervention-related sex differences in reducing depressive symptoms (Cuijpers et al., 2014).

Note on the Evidence Bearing on Burnout

The evidence on the efficacy of individual treatments for reducing symptoms of burnout has been much sparser and of lower quality (e.g., Tamminga et al., 2023) than the evidence bearing on individual treatments for depression. Given the overlap—notably, the symptom and etiological overlap—of burnout with depression, CBT and IPT designed to treat depressive conditions are likely to benefit individuals with burnout complaints.

Primary and Secondary Interventions for Depression, Psychological Distress, and Burnout

We now take a combined look at primary and secondary interventions because single meta-analyses involving interventions to address workplace stress tend to include both primary and secondary interventions (e.g., de Wijn & van der Doef, 2022; Panagioti et al., 2017; Richardson & Rothstein, 2008; West et al., 2016). However, with one exception, we limit ourselves to an examination of meta-analyses that exclusively comprise RCTs. Primary interventions theoretically address the sources of stress (e.g., improve work schedules). These interventions assume that job stress results from problematic work environments and attempt to reduce job stress by effecting change at the organizational level. Secondary interventions attempt to decrease stress-related symptoms before the symptoms worsen enough to jeopardize a person's health. Secondary interventions can be based on CBT or relaxation methods. CBT helps the individual reappraise a threatening work-related problem as more of a challenge than a threat and develop ways of coping with the challenge (Lazarus, 1995). Problem-solving is an important component of CBT. Relaxation techniques include progressive muscle relaxation, breathing exercises, yoga, and meditation. If an individual were highly symptomatic or met criteria for major depression, a tertiary psychotherapeutic intervention, such as CBT or IPT, would be called for.

Stress management interventions (SMIs) are programs that are often initiated by an organization's leadership, the purpose of which is to reduce the number or intensity of work-related stressors or minimize adverse consequences of workers' exposure to stressors (Richardson & Rothstein, 2008). These programs, the components of which are quite diverse, represent primary and secondary types of interventions. Many of the meta-analyses bearing on specific types of SMIs comprise fewer than ten RCTs. A threat to the validity of meta-analyses having statistically significant results that favor interventions but are based on few RCTs is that the findings could reflect the file drawer problem that we discussed earlier.

The meta-analysis conducted by Richardson and Rothstein (2008) is a landmark study. To our knowledge, it was the first meta-analysis of SMIs that was limited exclusively to randomized primary and secondary interventions. Richardson and Rothstein assembled 36 studies representing 55 interventions, some of which applied to psychological outcomes; other outcomes were organizational (e.g., increased productivity) and physiological (e.g., lowered blood pressure). The outcome closest to depression was general mental health/psychological distress, which was largely assessed by the GHQ-12, a composite instrument that includes depressive symptoms (e.g., anhedonia, low self-worth, depressed mood, worries).

Table 5.1 summarizes key findings that bear on mental health outcomes in Richardson and Rothstein's (2008) meta-analysis. As shown in the table, the average effect of all the SMIs aimed at reducing mental health symptoms was medium. The one study that was based on CBT had a large effect size. The smallest effect size was found for organizational interventions (participatory goal-setting; coworker support groups). The SMIs that had multiple components, which often included a cognitive component, had, on average, a medium effect in reducing mental health symptoms. The effect of relaxation/mindfulness SMIs on general mental health was between low and medium. Two studies used burnout as an outcome; no average result specific to burnout was presented. Richardson and Rothstein's meta-analysis was a good beginning. Given the number of studies, conclusions are tentative.

Physicians are members of an occupational group that can be subject to considerable job stress. Because we can't look at every occupational group, we decided to spotlight meta-analytic research on a small number of occupations, including physicians. The job of medical doctors can be very demanding, with long hours, having to be "on call," and life-or-death decision-making. One meta-analysis (West et al., 2016)

Table 5.1 Meta-analyses of mental health effects of different stress management interventions.

Stress Management Intervention	k	d
Cognitive behavioral	1	−0.71*
Relaxation/mindfulness	5	−0.40*
Organizational	3	−0.17
Multimodal	5	−0.52
Alternative	2	−0.62*
Grand average	16	−0.44**

Note: Multimodal interventions involve different combinations of components such as cognitive, relaxation, assertiveness training, goal setting, and so forth. Alternative interventions include exercise, journaling, or coping skills training.
k = number of randomized controlled trials that used the stress management intervention.
d = the effect size (Cohen's d)
*$p < .05$; **$p < .001$. Adapted from Richardson and Rothstein (2008).

identified 15 RCTs. Twelve of them involved small groups of physicians who were assigned self-care training SMIs (e.g., learning coping strategies); three RCTs involved structural/organizational changes in work environments (e.g., shortened shifts).[6] The study team did not break out the findings by type of intervention, although there was some evidence (augmented by the results of longitudinal research) that structural/organizational changes lead to greater reductions in burnout symptoms than secondary interventions. West et al. found that in the 12 RCTs that assessed EE, experimental groups averaged a two-point reduction on the MBI's EE subscale. Although the effect size was not reported, the two-point reduction is very small and clinically insignificant in view of the scaling involved.

Perhaps a better study of the effect of SMIs on burnout in physicians was conducted by Panagioti et al. (2017). Their meta-analysis ($k = 20$) assessed the impact of two general types of interventions on burnout's core EE symptoms. One type of intervention was directed at individual

---

6 Narrowly, these three RCTs involved primary interventions; the meta-analysis, however, included them with the other interventions, which were secondary interventions.

physicians. These interventions included CBT, mindfulness-based programs, and so on. The other type of intervention was directed at the work environment, including the introduction of changes such as reductions in workload. The average impact over all the interventions was small ($d = -0.29$). However, compared to the individually directed interventions ($d = -0.18$), the organizational interventions ($d = -0.45$) saw, on average, a significantly larger reduction in symptoms.

A meta-analysis (Petrie et al., 2019) involving seven RCTs assessed the impact of interventions on mental-health symptom reduction in physicians. Six interventions "were delivered universally to any working physician," and one involved every working mother. The interventions mostly involved mindfulness training, psychoeducation, and CBT-oriented stress management. Outcome measures varied and included depressed mood, anxiety (one study), general psychological distress (GHQ-12), and a single item on suicidal ideation (the ninth item on the PHQ-9). In reporting the overall results, two studies were omitted; otherwise, the included interventions were linked to a medium-to-large statistically significant average symptom reduction ($d = -0.65$).[7] The two omitted RCTs used a two-item depression screen to indicate probable depression, but the intervention effect was nonsignificant. One of the omitted studies (Dyrbye et al., 2016) also examined the MBI and showed no statistically significant results for EE, DP, or PA. We hope to see meta-analyses involving physicians with larger numbers of RCTs in the future.

Nursing has been linked to abundant job-related stressors, including overwork, understaffing, patient death, lack of autonomy, intense emotional work, and problematic nurse–physician relationships, all of which can have a baleful impact on nurses (Schonfeld & Chang, 2017). Breaking with our policy of only examining meta-analytic results based on RCTs, we examined the results of de Wijn and van der Doef (2022), who, in their meta-analyses, combined RCTs (most of the studies) and quasi-experiments. The interventions included CBT and relaxation. The investigators found low-to-medium, statistically significant intervention effects in lowering burnout symptoms[8] ($g = -0.30; k = 33$), psychological distress ($g = -0.39; k = 28$), and depressive symptoms ($g = -0.31; k = 24$).

---

7 The research team did not include a negative sign for reduced symptoms but to be consistent with our reporting, we included it here and elsewhere.
8 Burnout was not broken out by EE, DP, and PA.

There were no significant differences in the effects based on the types of interventions in reducing symptoms. The research team found that compared to shorter treatments, treatments with longer durations tended to lead to greater symptom reductions. de Wijn and van der Doef also identified organization-directed interventions, but they were few in number, with three having, on average, a small but statistically significant effect on burnout symptoms ($g = -0.14$).

High-stress jobs have been subject to interventions. The meta-analyses conducted by Estevez Cores et al. (2021) comprised "individual-focused stress management, health, or wellness interventions" that were applied to workers employed in "high-stress" jobs (e.g., education, healthcare). The participants, however, were deemed to be healthy, in effect making the interventions primary interventions. Tertiary interventions were excluded; studies involving workers who had been diagnosed with a major illness were also excluded. The numbers of studies pertinent to the components of burnout (EE, DP, and PA) were small ($5 \leq k \leq 8$). As shown in Table 5.2, the research team found that CBT had statistically significant effects in reducing EE and DP symptoms; the effect on PA was not significant. The largest effect of CBT was of medium size, on EE. Relaxation/mindfulness interventions had significant beneficial effects on all three burnout components ($3 \leq k \leq 7$); the effects were small to medium. Multimodal (combined) treatments had no significant effects on EE ($k = 4$) or PA ($k = 3$).

Estevez Cores et al. (2021) also examined the impact of interventions on psychological distress as assessed with the GHQ-12. Again, the numbers of studies were small. Table 5.2 shows that CBT had a significant small-to-medium effect in reducing psychological distress and relaxation/mindfulness had a medium-to-large significant effect in lowering distress. There was a small number of multimodal interventions that on average had a significant beneficial but modest effect on GHQ-12 scores. The alternative interventions were too diverse to draw a general conclusion about the impact of any one type of intervention on the GHQ-12 or EE.

Teachers are members of a profession that is sometimes exposed to occupational stressors in the form of unhelpful administrators, student disrespect, and violence and its threat (Bloch, 1978; Schonfeld, 2006; Schonfeld & Feinman, 2012; Schonfeld et al., 2017). Iancu et al. (2018) identified RCTs designed to reduce burnout symptoms in teachers. We concentrate on the impact of the interventions on EE and PA because the

Table 5.2 Meta-analyses bearing on workers in high-stress jobs.

Stress management intervention	GHQ-12		EE		DP		PA	
	k	g	k	g	k	g	k	g
CBT	6	−0.38***	8	−0.42***	6	−0.26*	5	−0.11
Relaxation/mindfulness	3	−0.64***	7	−0.30*	3	−0.32*	5	0.32*
Multimodal	4	−0.23*	4	−0.04			3	0.19
Alternative	3	−0.48***	5	−0.33**				

Note: CBT refers to cognitive behavioral therapy; multimodal interventions involve different combinations of components such as exercise, focus on health improvement, virtual reality, and so forth. Alternative interventions include probiotics, biofeedback, journaling, physical exercise, and career management.
k = number of randomized controlled trials in each meta-analysis
g = effect size (Hedges's g)
GHQ-12 = General Health Questionnaire, a measure of psychological distress;
EE = the Emotional Exhaustion subscale of the Maslach Burnout Inventory (MBI);
DP = Depersonalization subscale of the MBI; PA = the personal accomplishment subscale of the MBI.
* $p < .05$; ** $p < .01$; *** $p < .001$. Adapted from Estevez Cores et al. (2021).

effects on DP were weak and statistically nonsignificant (see Table 5.3). The average effects of CBT and mindfulness/meditation in reducing EE symptoms were small but statistically significant.

Professional development entails training teachers in such skills as classroom management. The average effect of professional development on EE was interesting because it was considerably larger than the effect of CBT and mindfulness/meditation. The impact of professional development, however, was *not* statistically significant. The reason for the lack of statistical significance is that there was great variation in the impact of the professional development interventions, with at least one intervention being very helpful ($d = -1.03$) and the others not (as indirectly evidenced by two of them having little effect on PA). One intervention even had a harmful effect on EE ($d = 0.11$). Although this is anecdotal, the first author had for six years been a mathematics teacher in the New York City public school system; his memories of professional development meetings he attended, although these characteristics have, he hopes, changed, were that they were largely soporific and laden with clichés.

Table 5.3 The results of meta-analyses bearing on teachers.

Stress management intervention	EE		PA	
	k	d	k	d
CBT	5	−0.20*	5	0.17
Mindfulness/meditation	6	−0.31**	5	0.28*
Social-emotional	3	−0.04	2	0.08
Psychoeducational	3	−0.09	3	0.07
Social support	3	−0.12	3	0.27*
Professional development	4	−0.46	2	0.10

Note: CBT refers to cognitive behavioral therapy.
Results on depersonalization were omitted because they were not significant.
k = number of randomized controlled trials in each meta-analysis
g = effect size (Hedges's g)
EE = the Emotional Exhaustion subscale of the Maslach Burnout Inventory (MBI);
PA = the personal accomplishment subscale of the MBI.
* $p < .05$; ** $p < .01$. Adapted from Iancu et al. (2018).

Mindfulness/meditation and social support had a small statistically significant effect on increasing PA. Social support could help teachers accomplish educational goals because support can come in the form of interaction with competent peers. Professional development had a surprisingly weak, nonsignificant effect on PA; however, there were only two studies that looked at professional development's effect on PA. Given the paucity of research on reducing teacher burnout, more research on high-quality professional development interventions is needed.

Mental health providers are tasked with helping people who are experiencing mental health problems. Providers, of course, are not exempt from having their own mental health problems. Although there were uncontrolled studies in Dreison et al.'s (2018) meta-analysis, we concentrate on the 13 RCTs encompassing interventions to treat burnout symptoms. Ten of the 13 interventions were organization-directed coworker support groups and job training/education. Although the analysis did not distinguish the effects of the organizational and person-level interventions, the overall effect size based on 12 RCTs was small and nonsignificant.

Thoughts on Primary and Secondary Interventions

The meta-analyses we reviewed tended to show that interventions such as CBT and meditation/mindfulness/relaxation lead to reductions in depressive/distress and burnout symptoms. The magnitude of the effect sizes varied from small to almost-large. There were more secondary than primary interventions. Secondary CBT-based interventions that help workers interpret stressors differently and develop strategies to deal with stressors appear to be beneficial. Relaxation interventions may provide a little help to workers experiencing job-related distress.

Those secondary interventions, however, don't change objective workplace stressors such as lack of formal control over the tasks for which the worker is responsible, unreasonably heavy workloads, workplace violence and its threat, and the intrusiveness of job conditions that create difficulties balancing work and family life. More research on primary interventions is needed. In fact, it would be helpful to see more primary interventions that are directed at changing organizational conditions that cannot be changed by more subjective means (e.g., by modifying one's expectations or adopting different coping strategies). Of course, such primary interventions need to be rigorously evaluated for their impact on the mental and, indeed, physical health of workers.

Another concern is that the workers who participated in the previously mentioned primary and secondary intervention studies were largely professional. It would also be helpful if a new generation of primary and secondary interventions were geared to blue- and pink-collar workers and custodial staffs and agricultural workers. In addition, it would be important to study the extent to which interventions operate similarly among workers of different racial or ethnic groups.

A Pertinent Primary Intervention Study

We turn to an innovative field experiment that may stimulate future primary intervention research. Kossek et al. (2019) developed a study the purpose of which was to evaluate the impact of an intervention to reduce psychological distress and life stress among more than 1,500 direct-care workers (nursing assistants and nurses) employed at long-term care facilities in New England. The study had four characteristics worth underscoring. First, the study was a cRCT (described earlier in the chapter). Organizations, rather than individual workers, were randomized to intervention and control conditions ("practice as usual"), an accommodation to the organizational landscape. Second, the cRCT was double-blind with the observers and participants not knowing who was in the experimental or control conditions, a rare feature in intervention research on psychological outcomes. Employees at all the sites perceived that they were participating in a study underwritten by the National Institutes of Health. Third, the research team analyzed the outcomes on an intention-to-treat basis (described earlier in the chapter). Fourth, the employees targeted were part of an economic sector characterized by high rates of turnover.

Based on the job demands–resources model (described in Chapter 2), the intervention comprised two components designed to provide the workers greater resources. In an effort "to increase employee control over work time," one component involved creating a management–worker steering committee to develop ways to improve worker control over schedules (any changes had to be cost-neutral and ensure patient safety). The second component involved training managers to be more supportive of the workers and the families they care for when not on the job. Although the duration of the intervention was 4 months, the post-intervention data collection period lasted 18 months.

We summarize a few key findings as follows:

1. Participants in the experimental and control groups showed comparable declines in psychological distress (scale items include "hopeless" and "so sad that nothing could cheer you up") and perceived life stress (reduced self-confidence in handling personal problems; inability can't overcome difficulties that have piled up) from pre-test baseline levels during the 6-, 12-, and 18-month follow-up periods.
2. At 18 months the intervention had a statistically significant small-to-medium effect in reducing life stress in workers who had childcare obligations. The effect was reflected in the statistic Δ, a cousin of Cohen's d ($\Delta = 0.34$).

3. At 12 months the intervention had a significant beneficial small-to-medium effect on life stress ($\Delta = 0.35$) and a small beneficial effect on psychological distress ($\Delta = 0.25$) for workers who had eldercare obligations. No significant effects were found at 6 and 18 months.
4. At 12 months the intervention had a significant small-to-medium beneficial effect on life stress ($\Delta = 0.40$) for workers who had "sandwiched care" responsibilities (eldercare and childcare).

A factor that mitigated against finding larger effects was a floor effect, namely, that pre-test scores on the distress and the life stress measures were relatively low to begin with (possibly a reflection of the healthy worker effect described in Chapter 1), making statistically significant decrements less likely to materialize. But clearly, the most impactful effects were on employees who had eldercare responsibilities. An implication of the findings is that future interventions should be more differentiated, with some approaches tailored to workers with different kinds of non-work responsibilities (childcare, eldercare). Moreover, given that this economic sector experiences turnover, it would have been helpful to have a glimpse at "as treated" results.

Conclusions

The evidence reviewed in Chapter 3 shows that what many people regard as burnout is in fact a depressive condition. The evidence holds whether we conceive of both burnout and depression as continua or whether we conceive both as diagnoses. That evidence has implications for treatment given the research reviewed in this chapter. We refer specifically to evidence demonstrating the efficacy of tertiary interventions such as CBT and ITP in treating depression. Individuals who describe themselves as suffering from burnout should consider seeking treatment from licensed professionals who are trained in treating depression.

For a self-described sufferer of burnout, and for anyone else, a vacation is fine. We are not opposed to vacations. But a vacation is not enough for the sufferer. The exhaustion found in burnout/depression does not reflect a healthy fatigue from which a worker could easily recover through some well-deserved rest; that exhaustion emerges from the experience of helplessness and entrapment that unresolvable stress entails (Bianchi et al., 2022; Schonfeld & Chang, 2017). With these considerations in mind, CBT and IPT are reasonable, time-limited treatment options. Given tales circulating about individuals in psychoanalysis for 15 years, the time-limited character of CBT and IPT is an advantage. The evidence behind their efficacy is solid. Moreover, unlike pharmacotherapy, CBT and IPT have no identified side effects.

An organization's human resources or employee assistance department can refer workers suffering from high levels of depressive or burnout symptoms to providers offering tertiary interventions such as CBT and IPT. However, it is more likely that such workers will seek treatment on their own, given privacy concerns. Privacy over depression is an important concern in many occupations, especially that of physicians because of negative consequences for licensing (Schonfeld, 2018). One recommendation we make regarding human resources and employee assistance departments is that, unless the help-seeker is in danger of self-harm or harming others, files on the help-seeker should not be made available to management. We believe in the importance of reducing as far as possible the risk of discrimination against help-seekers.

The history of public health tells us that primary prevention efforts have protected the health of more people and saved more lives than any other type of health-related intervention. We refer to such public health accomplishments as the provision of safe drinking water, sanitation, and campaigns to inoculate populations against infectious diseases. Primary prevention can also play a role in mental health, including the mental health of workers.

In research on occupational stress, primary interventions concentrate on workers clustered in organizational units or entire organizations. Certain approaches to organization-based interventions hold promise. Historically, employer concerns over the health and safety of employees have been fragmented (Schill & Choosewood, 2013). Human resources or employee assistance departments offer health promotion (HP) services, for example, secondary intervention activities such as programs to help workers who adopt healthier diets. They also can be a source of referrals to outside psychotherapists. Other departments are concerned with organizational health and safety (OSH), with one department creating and monitoring work schedules, another concerning itself with building mechanics such as ventilation, another department with workplace sanitation, and so on.

A program developed by the National Institute of Occupational Health and Safety (NIOSH) emphasizes interventions that coordinate OSH and HP. The strategy is known as Total Worker Health® (TWH).[9] Given that the causes of psychological and medical disorders are multifactorial, and include socioeconomic, organizational, and personal factors, the idea behind TWH is that "evidence-based practices bearing on the physical and organizational facets of the workplace as well as the health behaviors of workers can be integrated and harnessed to advance workers' physical and mental health" (Schonfeld & Chang, 2017, p. 334). An advantage of this approach is that it can apply to blue-collar and white-collar (really any collar) workers. One ongoing TWH intervention involves correctional officers (Cherniack et al., 2024). That intervention has relied on the participation of the officers in developing it and seeing it evolve.

We also note that the intervention by Kossek et al. (2019) can serve as an example of a primary intervention, not so much to emulate, but to stimulate other investigators. Kossek et al. had a worker–management steering committee develop an intervention that would serve as the experimental condition. A lesson learned from that effort is the importance of tailoring the components of an intervention to desired outcomes. The intervention appeared to reduce psychological distress and life stress in workers who have caregiving responsibilities outside of work but not in workers without those responsibilities. The development of primary interventions tailored to a specific group of workers and the nature of the work they perform has the potential to produce mental health benefits. Although these primary interventions are not the only ideas that can shoulder future interventions designed to diminish the presence of job stressors that provoke psychological distress in workers, they can motivate future research on making workplaces less stressful.

---

[9] The U.S. Department of Health and Human Services, of which Centers for Disease Control and Prevention (CDC) is a unit, trademarked the name of the strategy. NIOSH is a unit of the CDC.

References

Bartlett, L., Martin, A., Neil, A. L., Memish, K., Otahal, P., Kilpatrick, M., & Sanderson, K. (2019). A systematic review and meta-analysis of workplace mindfulness training randomized controlled trials. *Journal of Occupational Health Psychology, 24*(1), 108–126. https://doi.org/10.1037/ocp0000146

Beck, A. T. (1997). The past and future of cognitive therapy. *Journal of Psychotherapy Practice & Research, 6*(4), 276–284.

Bianchi, R., Wac, K., Sowden, J. F., & Schonfeld, I. S. (2022). Burned-out with burnout? Insights from historical analysis. *Frontiers in Psychology, 13*, 993208. https://doi.org/10.3389/fpsyg.2022.993208

Bloch, A. M. (1978). Combat neurosis in inner-city schools. *American Journal of Psychiatry, 135*(10), 1189–1192. https://doi.org/10.1176/ajp.135.10.1189

Borenstein, M., Hedges, L. V., Higgins, J. P. T., & Rothstein, H. R. (2021). *Introduction to meta-analysis* (2nd ed.). Wiley.

Cherniack, M., Namazi, S., Brennan, M., Henning, R., Dugan, A., & El Ghaziri, M. (2024). A 16-year chronicle of developing a healthy workplace participatory program for Total Worker Health® in the Connecticut Department of Correction: The Health Improvement through Employee Control (HITEC) Program. *International Journal of Environmental Research and Public Health, 21*(2), 142. https://doi.org/10.3390/ijerph21020142.

Cipriani, A., Furukawa, T. A., Salanti, G., Chaimani, A., Atkinson, L. Z., Ogawa, Y., Leucht, S., Ruhe, H. G., Turner, E. H., Higgins, J. P. T., Egger, M., Takeshima, N., Hayasaka, Y., Imai, H., Shinohara, K., Tajika, A., Ioannidis, J. P. A., & Geddes, J. R. (2018). Comparative efficacy and acceptability of 21 antidepressant drugs for the acute treatment of adults with major depressive disorder: A systematic review and network meta-analysis. *Lancet, 391*(10128), 1357–1366. https://doi.org/10.1016/S0140-6736(17)32802-7

Cohen, J. (1988). *Statistical power analysis for the behavioral sciences* (2nd ed.). Lawrence Erlbaum Associates.

Cooper, C. L., & Kompier, M. A. J. (Eds.) (1999). *Preventing stress, improving productivity: European case studies in the workplace*. Routledge.

Craighead, W. E., Johnson, B. N., Carey, S., & Dunlop, B. W. (2015). Psychosocial treatments for major depressive disorder. In P. E. Nathan and J. M. Gorman (Eds.), *A guide to treatments that work* (pp. 381–408). Oxford University Press.

Cuijpers, P., Berking, M., Andersson, G., Quigley, L., Kleiboer, A., & Dobson, K. S. (2013). A meta-analysis of cognitive-behavioural therapy for adult depression, alone and in comparison with other treatments. *The Canadian Journal of Psychiatry / La Revue Canadienne de Psychiatrie, 58*(7), 376–385.

Cuijpers, P., Donker, T., Weissman, M. M., Ravitz, P., & Cristea, I. A. (2016). Interpersonal psychotherapy for mental health problems: A comprehensive meta-analysis. *American Journal of Psychiatry, 173*(7), 680–687. https://doi.org/10.1176/appi.ajp.2015.15091141

Cuijpers, P., Harrer, M., Miguel, C., Ciharova, M., & Karyotaki, E. (2023a). Five decades of research on psychological treatments of depression: A historical and meta-analytic overview. *American Psychologist*. https://doi.org/10.1037/amp0001250

Cuijpers, P., Karyotaki, E., Harrer, M., & Stikkelbroek, Y. (2023b). Individual behavioral activation in the treatment of depression: A meta analysis. *Psychotherapy Research, 33*(7), 886–897. https://doi.org/10.1080/10503307.2023.2197630

Cuijpers, P., Noma, H., Karyotaki, E., Cipriani, A., & Furukawa, T. A. (2019). Effectiveness and acceptability of cognitive behavior therapy delivery formats in adults with depression: A network meta-analysis. *JAMA Psychiatry, 76*(7), 700–707. https://doi.org/10.1001/jamapsychiatry.2019.0268

Cuijpers, P., Noma, H., Karyotaki, E., Vinkers, C. H., Cipriani, A., & Furukawa, T. A. (2020). A network meta-analysis of the effects of psychotherapies, pharmacotherapies and their combination in the treatment of adult depression. *World Psychiatry, 19*(1), 92–107. https://doi.org/10.1002/wps.20701

Cuijpers, P., Weitz, E., Twisk, J., Kuehner, C., Cristea, I., David, D., DeRubeis, R. J., Dimidjian, S., Dunlop, B. W., Faramarzi, M., Hegerl, U., Jarrett, R. B., Kennedy, S. H., Kheirkhah, F., Mergl, R., Miranda, J., Mohr, D. C., Segal, Z. V., Siddique, J., . . . Hollon, S. D. (2014). Gender as predictor and moderator of outcome in cognitive behavior therapy and pharmacotherapy for adult depression: An "individual patient data" meta-analysis. *Depression and Anxiety, 31*(11), 941–951. https://doi.org/10.1002/da.22328

de Wijn, A. N., & van der Doef, M. P. (2022). A meta-analysis on the effectiveness of stress management interventions for nurses: Capturing 14 years of research. *International Journal of Stress Management, 29*(2), 113–129. https://doi.org/10.1037/str0000169

Dettori, J. R., Norvell, D. C., & Chapman, J. R. (2022). Fixed-effect vs random-effects models for meta-analysis: 3 points to consider. *Global Spine Journal, 12*(7), 1624–1626. https://doi.org/10.1177/21925682221110527

Dimidjian, S., Barrera, M., Jr., Martell, C., Muñoz, R. F., & Lewinsohn, P. M. (2011). The origins and current status of behavioral activation treatments for depression. *Annual Review of Clinical Psychology, 7*, 1–38. https://doi.org/10.1146/annurev-clinpsy-032210-104535

Dreison, K. C., Luther, L., Bonfils, K. A., Sliter, M. T., McGrew, J. H., & Salyers, M. P. (2018). Job burnout in mental health providers: A meta-analysis of 35 years of intervention research. *Journal of Occupational Health Psychology, 23*(1), 18–30. https://doi.org/10.1037/ocp0000047

Dyrbye, L. N., West, C. P., Richards, M. L., Ross, H. J., Satele, D., & Shanafelt, T. D. (2016). A randomized, controlled study of an online intervention to promote job satisfaction and well-being among physicians. *Burnout Research, 3*(3), 69–75. https://doi.org/10.1016/j.burn.2016.06.002

Estevez Cores, S., Sayed, A. A., Tracy, D. K., & Kempton, M. J. (2021). Individual-focused occupational health interventions: A meta-analysis of randomized controlled trials. *Journal of Occupational Health Psychology, 26*(3), 189–203. https://doi.org/10.1037/ocp0000249

Furukawa, T. A., Weitz, E. S., Tanaka, S., Hollon, S. D., Hofmann, S. G., Andersson, G., Twisk, J., DeRubeis, R. J., Dimidjian, S., Hegerl, U., Mergl, R., Jarrett, R. B., Vittengl, J. R., Watanabe, N., & Cuijpers, P. (2017). Initial severity of depression and efficacy of cognitive–behavioural therapy: Individual-participant data meta-analysis of pill-placebo-controlled trials. *British Journal of Psychiatry, 210*(3), 190–196. https://doi.org/10.1192/bjp.bp.116.187773

Grossman, P. (2015). Mindfulness: Awareness informed by an embodied ethic. *Mindfulness, 6*(1), 17–22. https://doi.org/10.1007/s12671-014-0372-5

Haslam, A., Tuia, J., Miller, S. L., & Prasad, V. (2023). Systematic review and meta-analysis of randomized trials testing interventions to reduce physician burnout. *American Journal of Medicine, 137*(3), 249–257. https://doi.org/10.1016/j.amjmed.2023.10.003

Hayes, S. C., Luoma, J. B., Bond F. W., Masuda, A., & Lillis, J. (2006). Acceptance and commitment therapy: Model, processes and outcomes. *Behavioural Research and Therapy, 44* (1), 1–25. https://doi.org/10.1016/j.brat.2005.06.006

Hedges, L. V., & Olkin, I. (1985). *Statistical methods for meta-analysis*. Academic Press.

Iancu, A. E., Rusu, A., Măroiu, C., Păcurar, R., & Maricuțoiu, L. P. (2018). The effectiveness of interventions aimed at reducing teacher burnout: A meta-analysis. *Educational Psychology Review, 30*(2), 373–396. https://doi.org/10.1007/s10648-017-9420-8

Ijaz, S., Davies, P., Williams, C. J., Kessler, D., Lewis, G., & Wiles, N. (2018). Psychological therapies for treatment-resistant depression in adults. *Cochrane Database of Systematic Reviews* (5), CD010558. https://doi.org/10.1002/14651858.CD010558.pub2

Joyce, S., Modini, M., Christensen, H., Mykletun, A., Bryant, R., Mitchell, P. B., & Harvey, S. B. (2016). Workplace interventions for common mental disorders: A systematic meta-review. *Psychological Medicine, 46*(4), 683–697. https://doi.org/10.1017/S0033291715002408

Kellogg, S. H., & Young, J. E. (2008). Cognitive therapy. In J. L. Lebow (Ed.), *Twenty-first century psychotherapies* (pp. 43–79). Wiley.

Kossek, E. E., Thompson, R. J., Lawson, K. M., Bodner, T., Perrigino, M. B., Hammer, L. B., Buxton, O. M., Almeida, D. M., Moen, P., Hurtado, D. A., Wipfli, B., Berkman, L. F., & Bray, J. W. (2019). Caring for the elderly at work and home: Can a randomized organizational intervention improve psychological health? *Journal of Occupational Health Psychology, 24*(1), 36–54. https://doi.org/10.1037/ocp0000104

Kühnel, J., & Sonnentag, S. (2011). How long do you benefit from vacation? A closer look at the fade-out of vacation effects. *Journal of Organizational Behavior, 32*(11), 125–143. http://dx.doi.org/10.1002/job.699

Lazarus, R. S. (1995). Psychological stress in the workplace. In *Occupational stress: A handbook* (pp. 3–14). Taylor & Francis.

Li, X.- M., Huang, F.- F., Cuijpers, P., Liu, H., Karyotaki, E., Li, Z.- J., Miguel, C., Ciharova, M., & Dobson, K. (2024). The efficacy of cognitive behavioral therapies for depression in China in comparison with the rest of the world: A systematic review and meta-analysis. *Journal of*

Consulting and Clinical Psychology, 92(2), 105–117. https://doi.org/10.1002/cpp.1774

Ljótsson, B., Hedman, E., Mattsson, S., & Andersson, E. (2015). The effects of cognitive–behavioral therapy for depression are not falling: A re-analysis of Johnsen and Friborg (2015). *Psychological Bulletin, 143*(3), 321–325. https://doi.org/10.1037/bul0000055

Lucas, B. P., Trick, W. E., Evans, A. T., Mba, B., Smith, J., Das, K., Clarke, P., Varkey, A., Mathew, S., & Weinstein, R. A. (2012). Effects of 2- vs 4-week attending physician inpatient rotations on unplanned patient revisits, evaluations by trainees, and attending physician burnout: A randomized trial. *JAMA, 308*(21), 2199–2207. https://doi.org/10.1001/jama.2012.36522

Markowitz, J. C., & Weissman, M. M. (2004). Interpersonal psychotherapy: Principles and applications. *World Psychiatry, 3*(3), 136–139.

Markowitz, J. C., & Weissman, M. M. (2012). Interpersonal psychotherapy: Past, present and future. *Clinical Psychology & Psychotherapy, 19*(2), 99–105. https://doi.org/10.1002/cpp.1774

Miao, C., Gao, Y., Li, X., Zhou, Y., Chung, J. W.-Y., & Smith, G. D. (2023). The effectiveness of mindfulness yoga on patients with major depressive disorder: a systematic review and meta-analysis of randomized controlled trials. *BMC Complementary Medicine and Therapies, 23*(1), 3–13. https://doi.org/10.1186/s12906-023-04141-2

Oral, M., & Karakurt, N. (2024). The effectiveness of group interpersonal therapy on burnout among long-term care workers. *International Journal of Older People Nursing, 19*(5), e12639. https://doi.org/10.1111/opn.12639

Orwin, R. G. (1983). A fail-safe N for effect size in meta-analysis. *Journal of Educational Statistics, 8*(2), 157–159. https://doi.org/10.2307/1164923

Panagioti, M., Panagopoulou, E., Bower, P., Lewith, G., Kontopantelis, E., Chew-Graham, C., Dawson, S., van Marwijk, H., Geraghty, K., & Esmail, A. (2017). Controlled interventions to reduce burnout in physicians: A systematic review and meta-analysis. *JAMA Internal Medicine, 177*(2), 195–205. https://doi.org/10.1001/jamainternmed.2016.7674

Petrie, K., Crawford, J., Baker, S. T. E., Dean, K., Robinson, J., Veness, B. G., Randall, J., McGorry, P., Christensen, H., & Harvey, S. B. (2019). Interventions to reduce symptoms of common mental disorders and suicidal ideation in physicians: A systematic review and meta-analysis.

Lancet Psychiatry, 6(3), 225–234. https://doi.org/10.1016/s2215-0366 (18)30509-1

Prudenzi, A., Graham, C. D., Clancy, F., Hill, D., O'Driscoll, R., Day, F., & O'Connor, D. B. (2021). Group-based acceptance and commitment therapy interventions for improving general distress and work-related distress in healthcare professionals: A systematic review and meta-analysis. *Journal of Affective Disorders, 295,* 192–202. https://doi.org/10.1016/j.jad.2021.07.084

Punnett, L., Cavallari, J. M., Henning, R. A., Nobrega, S., Dugan, A. G., & Cherniack, M. G. (2020). Defining "Integration" for Total Worker Health®: A new proposal. *Annals of Work Exposures and Health, 64*(3), 223–235. https://doi.org/10.1093/annweh/wxaa003

Ren, Z., Zhao, C., Bian, C., Zhu, W., Jiang, G., & Zhu, Z. (2019). Mechanisms of the acceptance and commitment therapy: A meta-analytic structural equation model. *Acta Psychologica Sinica, 51*(6), 662–676. https://doi.org/10.3724/SP.J.1041.2019.00662

Richardson, K. M., & Rothstein, H. R. (2008). Effects of occupational stress management intervention programs: A meta-analysis. *Journal of Occupational Health Psychology, 13*(1), 69–93. https://doi.org/10.1037/1076-8998.13.1.69

Riegelman, R. K. (2005). *Studying a study and testing a test* (5th ed.). Lippincott Williams & Wilkins.

Rosenthal, R. (1979). The file drawer problem and tolerance for null results. *Psychological Bulletin, 86*(3), 638–641. https://doi.org/10.1037/0033-2909.86.3.638

Schill, A. L., & Chosewood, L. C. (2013). The NIOSH Total Worker Health™ program: An overview. *Journal of Occupational and Environmental Medicine, 55*(12 Suppl.), S8–S11. https://doi.org/10.1097/JOM.0000000000000037

Schmidt, L. R. (1994). A psychological look at public health: Contents and methodology. In S. Maes, H. Leventhal, & M. Johnston (Eds.), *International review of health psychology* (Vol. 3, pp. 3–36). Wiley.

Schonfeld, I. S. (2006). School violence. In E.K. Kelloway, J. Barling, & J.J. Hurrell, Jr. (Eds.), *Handbook of workplace violence* (pp. 169–229). Sage Publications. https://doi.org/10.4135/9781412976947.n9

Schonfeld, I. S. (2018, July 3). When we say "physician burnout," we really mean depression. *Medscape Psychiatry.* https://www.medscape.com/viewarticle/898662

Schonfeld, I. S., Bianchi, R., & Luehring-Jones, P. (2017). Consequences of job stress for the psychological well-being of teachers. In T. M. McIntyre, S. E. McIntyre, & D. J. Francis (Eds.), *Educator stress: An occupational health perspective* (pp. 55–75). Springer International Publishing. https://doi.org/10.1007/978-3-319-53053-6_3

Schonfeld, I. S., & Chang, C.-H. (2017). *Occupational health psychology: Work, stress, and health*. Springer Publishing Company. https://doi.org/10.1891/9780826199683

Schonfeld, I. S., & Feinman, S. J. (2012). Difficulties of alternatively certified teachers. *Education and Urban Society, 44*(3), 215–246. https://doi.org/10.1177/0013124510392570

Schramm, E., Mack, S., Thiel, N., Jenkner, C., Elsaesser, M., & Fangmeier, T. (2020). Interpersonal psychotherapy vs. treatment as usual for major depression related to work stress: A pilot randomized controlled study. *Frontiers in Psychiatry, 11*(193). https://doi.org/10.3389/fpsyt.2020.00193

Sekhar, P., Tee, Q. X., Ashraf, G., Trinh, D., Shachar, J., Jiang, A., Hewitt, J., Green, S., & Turner, T. (2021). Mindfulness-based psychological interventions for improving mental well-being in medical students and junior doctors. *Cochrane Database of Systematic Reviews* (12), CD013740. https://doi.org/10.1002/14651858.CD013740.pub2

Sullivan, H. S. (1953). *The interpersonal theory of psychiatry*. Norton.

Tamminga, S. J., Emal, L. M., Boschman, J. S., Levasseur, A., Thota, A., Ruotsalainen, J. H., Schelvis, R. M. C., van Nieuwenhuijsen, K., & der Molen, H. F. (2023). Individual-level interventions for reducing occupational stress in healthcare workers. *Cochrane Database of Systematic Reviews* (5), CD002892. https://doi.org/10.1002/14651858.CD002892.pub6

VandenBos, G. R. (2015). *APA dictionary of psychology* (2nd ed.). American Psychological Association. https://doi.org/10.1037/14646-000

Virgili, M. (2015). Mindfulness-based interventions reduce psychological distress in working adults: A meta-analysis of intervention studies. *Mindfulness, 6*(2), 326–337. https://doi.org/10.1007/s12671-013-0264-0

Weissman, M. M., Markowitz, J. C., & Klerman, G. L. (2018). *The guide to interpersonal psychotherapy* (Updated and expanded ed.). Oxford University Press.

West, C. P., Dyrbye, L. N., Erwin, P. J., & Shanafelt, T. D. (2016). Interventions to prevent and reduce physician burnout: A systematic review and meta-analysis. *Lancet, 388*(10057), 2272–2281. https://doi.org/10.1016/S0140-6736(16)31279-X

Westman, M., & Eden, D. (1997). Effects of a respite from work on burnout: Vacation relief and fade-out. *Journal of Applied Psychology, 82*(4), 516–527. https://doi.org/10.1037/0021-9010.82.4.516

Westman, M., & Etzion, D. (2001). The impact of vacation and job stress on burnout and absenteeism. *Psychology & Health, 16*(5), 595–606. https://doi.org/10.1080/08870440108405529

Xu, H., Cai, J., Sawhney, R., Jiang, S., Buys, N., & Sun, J. (2024). The effectiveness of cognitive-behavioral therapy in helping people on sick leave to return to work: A systematic review and meta-analysis. *Journal of Occupational Rehabilitation, 34*(1), 4–36. https://doi.org/10.1007/s10926-023-10116-4

Appendix

Occupational Depression Inventory (ODI)

Preliminary Instructions to Respondents

The following statements concern the impact your work could have had on you.

Please read each statement and indicate how often you experienced the problems mentioned over the PAST TWO WEEKS. Use the scale provided to respond:

0 = never or almost never
1 = a few days only
2 = more than half the days
3 = nearly every day

Here is an example:
"I felt anxious because of my job."

- If you did NOT feel anxious because of your job, select 0.
- If you felt anxious for reasons that are UNCONNECTED TO YOUR JOB (personal problems, marital problems, family problems, health problems, etc.), select 0 as well.
- If you felt anxious but don't know why, again select 0.
- If it is clear for you that YOUR JOB caused you to feel anxious, select 1, 2 or 3 to indicate how often that happened.

You can now complete the questionnaire.

Occupational Depression Inventory (ODI)

Patient name:.................................... Date:....................................

Indicate how often you experienced the problems mentioned below over the past two weeks.	Never or almost never	A few days only	More than half the days	Nearly every day
1. My work was so stressful that I could not enjoy the things that I usually like doing.	0	1	2	3
2. I felt depressed because of my job.	0	1	2	3
3. The stress of my job caused me to have sleep problems (I had difficulties falling asleep or staying asleep, or I slept much more than usual).	0	1	2	3
4. I felt exhausted because of my work.	0	1	2	3
5. I felt my appetite was disturbed because of the stress of my job (I lost my appetite, or the opposite, I ate too much).	0	1	2	3
6. My experience at work made me feel like a failure.	0	1	2	3
7. My job stressed me so much that I had trouble focusing on what I was doing (e.g., reading a newspaper article) or thinking clearly (e.g., to make decisions).	0	1	2	3
8. As a result of job stress, I felt restless, or the opposite, noticeably slowed down—for example, in the way I moved or spoke.	0	1	2	3
9. I thought that I'd rather be dead than continue in this job.	0	1	2	3

TOTAL SCORE: ....

If you have encountered at least some of the problems mentioned above, do these problems lead you to consider leaving your current job or position?

☐ Yes ☐ No ☐ I don't know

Inventaire de Dépression Professionnelle (IDP)

Instructions Préliminaires Aux Répondants

Les propositions suivantes concernent l'impact que votre travail aurait pu avoir sur vous.

Veuillez lire chaque proposition et indiquer à quelle fréquence vous avez rencontré les problèmes mentionnés au cours des DEUX DERNIÈRES SEMAINES. Utilisez l'échelle fournie pour répondre:

0 = jamais ou presque jamais
1 = quelques jours seulement
2 = plus de la moitié du temps
3 = tous les jours ou presque

Voici un exemple:
"Je me suis senti(e) anxieux/se à cause de mon travail."

- Si vous NE vous êtes PAS senti(e) anxieux/se à cause de votre travail, sélectionnez 0.
- Si vous vous êtes senti(e) anxieux/se pour des raisons qui sont SANS LIEN AVEC VOTRE TRAVAIL (problèmes personnels, conjugaux, familiaux, de santé, etc.), sélectionnez également 0.
- Si vous vous êtes senti(e) anxieux/se mais ne savez pas pourquoi, de nouveau sélectionnez 0.
- S'il est clair pour vous que VOTRE TRAVAIL vous a rendu anxieux/se, sélectionnez 1, 2 ou 3 pour indiquer à quelle fréquence cela s'est produit.

Vous pouvez maintenant répondre au questionnaire.

Inventaire de Dépression Professionnelle (IDP)

Nom du patient: .... Date: ....

Indiquez à quelle fréquence vous avez fait l'expérience des problèmes évoqués ci-dessous au cours des deux dernières semaines.	Jamais ou presque jamais	Quelques jours seulement	Plus de la moitié du temps	Tous les jours ou presque
1. Mon travail a été si stressant que je n'arrivais pas à profiter des choses qui d'habitude me font plaisir.	0	1	2	3
2. Je me suis senti(e) déprimé(e) à cause de mon travail.	0	1	2	3
3. J'ai senti que mon sommeil était perturbé à cause de problèmes liés à mon travail (j'ai éprouvé des difficultés à m'endormir ou à rester endormi(e), ou au contraire j'ai dormi beaucoup plus que d'habitude).	0	1	2	3
4. Je me suis senti(e) épuisé(e) à cause de mon travail.	0	1	2	3
5. J'ai senti que mon appétit était perturbé à cause du stress lié à mon travail (j'ai perdu l'appétit, ou au contraire j'ai mangé beaucoup plus que d'habitude).	0	1	2	3
6. Je me suis senti(e) en échec personnel à cause de mon travail.	0	1	2	3

Inventaire de Dépression Professionnelle (IDP)

Nom du patient: .... Date: ....

Indiquez à quelle fréquence vous avez fait l'expérience des problèmes évoqués ci-dessous au cours des deux dernières semaines.	*Jamais ou presque jamais*	*Quelques jours seulement*	*Plus de la moitié du temps*	*Tous les jours ou presque*
7. Mon travail m'a stressé(e) à tel point que j'ai eu du mal à me concentrer sur ce que je faisais (par exemple, lire la presse) ou à penser clairement (par exemple, pour prendre des décisions).	0	1	2	3
8. À cause du stress lié à mon travail, je me suis senti(e) sensiblement agité(e), ou au contraire sensiblement ralenti(e) – par exemple dans ma façon de bouger ou de parler.	0	1	2	3
9. Je me suis dit que je préférerais être mort(e) plutôt que de continuer dans ce travail.	0	1	2	3

SCORE TOTAL: ....

Si vous avez rencontré au moins certains des problèmes évoqués ci-dessus, ces problèmes vous amènent-ils à envisager de quitter votre emploi ou poste actuel ?

☐ Oui   ☐ Non   ☐ Je ne sais pas

Index

Note: Page numbers in *italics* and **bold** refers to figures and tables respectively.

a

Abraham, Karl 5
Administrative Science Quarterly (Karasek) 27
Ahola, K. 117, 132
alienation 13
The Anatomy of Melancholy (Burton) 4
anxiety 18
  in burnout-depression overlap 124–127, **125**
Aronsson, G. 94, 95–96, 102
atherogenesis 30
attributional styles 11

b

Bahlmann, J. 156
Bakker, A. B. 87., 115
Beck, Aaron 8–9, 174–175
beck depression inventory (BDI) 87
behavioral activation (BA) 178

Bianchi, R. 21, 85, 93, 105, 116–121, 122, 126, 130, 131, 135, 157, 160, 192
Bibring, Edward 29
Borenstein, M. 172
Bradley, H. B. 73
Brown, George W. 22, 23, 81, 72, 85
burnout 156–159
  antecedents of 88–89
  Aronsson, G. (2017) 94, 95–96
  correlation coefficients 78–80
  destigmatizing 159–160
  as diagnosis 93–94
  discriminant validity 87–88
  evidence bearing on 182
  foundations of 80–86, **84, 86**
  Freudenberger, Herbert J. 74–76
  Guthier, C. (2020) 100–102
  Lesener, T. (2019) 96–99, **97, 99**
  longitudinal research on adverse working conditions and 94

burnout (*continued*)
    Maslach, Christina 76–78
    meta-analyses' findings 102–103
    multiplication of 89–92
    primary and secondary interventions for 182–189, **184, 187**
    problems with 92–93
    reliability coefficients 78–80
burnout–depression overlap 113–114
    anxiety symptoms 124–127, **125**
    as distinct constructs 114–116
    and depressive cognition 121–122
    depressive symptoms 124–127, **125**
    line of research 116–121, **118, 119**
    meta-analyses 133–137, **133, 134, 135, 137**
    neurobiology of 123–124
    occupational depression inventory (ODI) 127–131, **129, 130**
    studies 131–132
    syndrome, idea of 113
A Burnt-Out Case (Greene) 73
Burton, Robert 4
Buunk, B. P. 117

c

Calixto Cavalcante, D. 131, 135
cardiovascular disease (CVD) 32
Center for Epidemiologic Studies Depression Scale (CES-D) 54, 87–88
Chang, C. -H. 90–91

Child Youth Care Forum (Pines) 77
cognitive behavioral therapy (CBT) 167, 174–175
    thoughts on 181
confirmatory factor analysis (CFA) 87, 120, 130
conservation of resources (COR) theory 91
construct validity of burnout scales 114
continuum of depression 17–18, *18*
convergent validity of psychological scale 115
Copenhagen Burnout Inventory (CBI) 91, 129
correlation coefficients 78–80
cortisol 123–124
Cuijpers, P. 176, 181

d

De Beer, L. T. 126–127
decision latitude 29
demand–control (DC) model of job stress 27–31, **29**, 45
demand–control–support (DCS) model of job stress 32–33, **34–44**
Demerouti, E. 90
depersonalization (DP) 82
depression 156–159
    as distinct constructs 114–116
    neurobiology of 123–124
    primary and secondary interventions for 182–189, **184, 187**
    depressive cognition, burnout and 121–122

depressive symptoms, in burnout-depression overlap 124–127, **125**
Diagnostic and Statistical Manual (DSM-5) 15, 17
dichotomy 123
discriminant validity of burnout scales 87–88, 115
The Division of Labor in Society (Durkheim) 13
Dohrenwend, Barbara Snell 22, 33
Dohrenwend, Bruce 33
Dreison, K. C. 188
drift hypothesis 100
Durkheim, Émile 13–14, 32
Durup, J. 115

e
effort-reward imbalance (ERI) model 45–47, **48–52**
Ellis, Albert 8, 174
emotional exhaustion (EE) 82, 113
Enzmann, D. 88–89
The Epic of Gilgamesh 1
error, in psychometric theory 80
Estevez Cores, S. 186, **187**
exhaustion factor 121
exploratory structural equation modeling (ESEM) bifactor analysis 126

f
Freud, Sigmund 4–6
explanation of depression 6–9
Freudenberger, Herbert J. 74–76, 80–81, 103, 114

g
Gardell, Bertil 29
Ginsburg, Sigmund G. 73
Greene, Graham 73
Guthier, C. 94, 100–102, 103, 104, 112

h
HARKing (Hypothesizing After the Results are Known) 102
Harris, Tirril 22, 23, 72, 85
helplessness theory of depression 10–11, 122
Hempel, Carl 72
high-stress jobs 186
hippocratic humoral theory of melancholia 4
Holmes, Thomas H. 21–22
hopelessness theory of depression 10–11
Human Behavior: The Newsmagazine of the Social Sciences (Maslach) 76
Human Relations (journal) 28
Hurvich, Marvin 8
hypercortisolism 123
hypocortisolism 123

i
Iancu, A. E. 186, **188**
Ijaz, S. 177
An Inquiry into the Nature and Causes of the Wealth of Nations (Smith) 12
International Classification of Diseases 17
interpersonal therapy (IPT), 167, 179
thoughts on 181

interventions
  meta-analyses 168–173
  models of 165–168
  pertinent primary intervention study 189–191
  primary interventions 182–189, **184**, **187**
  randomized control trials (RCTs), 168–173
  secondary interventions 182–189, **184**, **187**
  success of 167
  tertiary interventions 173–182

j

Jackson, S. E., 82–83, 85–86
Jackson, Susan 81
Jahoda, Marie 15
job demands–resources (JD–R) model 90, 96
job stress
  demand–control (DC) model of 27–31, **29**
  demand–control–support (DCS) model of 32–33, **34–44**
Johnson, J. V. 32
Journal of Occupational Behaviour (Maslach and Jackson) 81
Journal of Social Issues (Freudenberger) 74, 78, 114

k

Karasek, Robert 27–31, **29**, 32, 33
Kim, S. 135
Klerman, Gerald L. 179
Kossek, E. E. 169, 170, 189
Koutsimani, P. 133, 135
Kraepelin, Emil 4
Kristensen, T. S. 91

l

Laurent, E. 116, 122
Leiter, M. P. 87–88, 93, 115, 120
Lesener, T. 94, 96–99, **97**, **99**, 103
Lucas, B. P. 169

m

Maier, Steven F. 10
major depressive disorder (MDD) 15–16
manic-depressive psychosis 4
Marienthal: The Sociography of an Unemployed Community (Jahoda) 15
Martin, Douglas 74
Marx, Karl 12–13
Maslach, Christina 76–78, 80–83, 85, **86**, 88, 93, 103, 112, 113, 114, 117, 120, 157, 159, 160
Maslach Burnout Inventory (MBI) 81–93, 103, 104, 112, 113–122, 124, 125, 127–130, 132–136, 139, 184, 185, 187, 188
MBI-General Survey (MBI-GS) 90, 117, 128–129
Meier, S. T. 84, 90, 114, 115, 135
Melamed, S. 91
melancholia 4
Melnick, E. R. 111
Mendel, R. 157
meta-analyses 168–173, 183, 185
  of burnout–depression overlap 133–137, **133**, **134**, **135**, **137**
Meyer, Adolf 4, 179
mindfulness therapy 178–179

n

neuroticism 43, 88
nomological network 119, 121, 126, 138

o

occupational depression
  as continuum 17–18, *18*
  demand–control (DC) model of job stress 27–31, **29**
  demand–control–support (DCS) model of job stress 32–33, **34–44**
  diagnosis of 15–17
  effort–reward imbalance (ERI) model **34–44**, 45–47, **48–52**
  Freud's explanation, challenge to 6–9
  helplessness 10–11
  history of 1–5
  hopelessness 10–11
  rage turned inward 5–6
  in research context 19
  reverse causality 33, 45
  stressful life events 21–27, *26*, **34–44, 48–52**
  The Stress of Life 19–21
  underestimates 53–55
  workplace bullying 47, 53
  work to psychological state, early linkages of 11–15
occupational depression inventory (ODI) 127–131, **129, 130**
occupational health psychology (OHP) 165
Oldenburg Burnout Inventory (OLBI) 90
Oswin, Maureen 21

p

Panagioti, M. 169, 184
Parkes, Katharine 20–21
passive jobs 31
personal accomplishment (PA) 82
pertinent primary intervention study 189–191
Pines, Ayala 77, 78, 83, 85, 89, 114
Popper, Karl 6–7
primary intervention 166, 182–189, **184, 187**
Prudenzi, A. 176
psychological distress, primary and secondary interventions for 182–189, **184, 187**
psychotherapy 173
Psychotherapy: Theory, Research and Practice (Freudenberger) 74
public stigma 153

r

Rahe, Richard H. 21–22
Ramazzini, Bernardino 11–12
randomized control trials (RCTs) 168–173
refuge hypothesis 100
reliability coefficients 78–80
reverse causality 33, 45
Richardson, K. M. 167, 183, **184**
Rosenthal, Robert 172
Rössler, W. 132
Rotenstein, L. S. 94, 96, 117
Rothstein, H. R. 167, 183

s

Schaufeli, W. B. 85, 88–89, 112, 117

Schonfeld, I. S.   12, 18, 20, 21, 24–25, **26,** 30, 32, 33, 45, 47, 90–91, 116–121, 130, 133, 135, 165, 166, 168, 185, 186, 192, 193
secondary intervention   166–167, 182–189, **184, 187**
self-stigma   153–154
Seligman, Martin E.   10
Selye, Hans   19–20
Sen, S.   159
Shirom, A.   91
Shirom-Melamed Burnout Measure (SMBM)   91, 118
Siegrist, Johannes   46–47
Smith, Adam   12
Smith, J.   158
The Social Origins of Depression (Brown and Harris)   22–24, 180
social readjustment rating scale (SRRS)   21–22
Sommer, Robert   73
Sowden, J.   130–131, 135–136
Staff Burn-Out (Freudenberger)   74–75
Sterkens, P.   155
stigma
  background beliefs   154
  burnout,
    destigmatizing   159–160
  burnout *vs.* depression   156–159
  empirical research   155–156
stressful life events (SLEs)   21–27, *26,* 33, **34–44, 48–52**

stress management interventions (SMIs)   182–183
The Stress of Life   19–21
stressor creation hypothesis   100
stressor perception hypothesis   100
suicidal ideation   4, 6, 14, 93, 118–119, 127, 129, 147, 185
suicide   13–14, 16, 32, 77, 93, 118–119, 127, 141
Sullivan, Harry Stack   179
Swingler, G.   136
Syndromal hypothesis   86, 104, 113–116, 121, 124, 126, 129, 131, 133–136, 138–140, 154

t

tertiary interventions   167, 173
  burnout, evidence bearing on   182
  IPT and CBT, thoughts on   181

v

Verkuilen, J.   121

w

Weissman, Myrna M.   179–180
West, C. P.   184
workplace bullying   47, 53
work to psychological state, early linkages of   11–15
Wurm, W.   131

x

Xu, H.   177